This report contains the collective views of an international group of experts and does not necessarily represent the decisions or the stated policy of the United Nations Environment Programme, the International Labour Organisation, or the World Health Organization.

Environmental Health Criteria 107

BARIUM

Published under the joint sponsorship of
the United Nations Environment Programme,
the International Labour Organisation,
and the World Health Organization

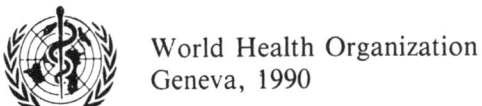

World Health Organization
Geneva, 1990

The **International Programme on Chemical Safety** (IPCS) is a joint venture of the United Nations Environment Programme, the International Labour Organisation, and the World Health Organization. The main objective of the IPCS is to carry out and disseminate evaluations of the effects of chemicals on human health and the quality of the environment. Supporting activities include the development of epidemiological, experimental laboratory, and risk-assessment methods that could produce internationally comparable results, and the development of manpower in the field of toxicology. Other activities carried out by the IPCS include the development of know-how for coping with chemical accidents, coordination of laboratory testing and epidemiological studies, and promotion of research on the mechanisms of the biological action of chemicals.

WHO Library Cataloguing in Publication Data

Barium.

(Environmental health criteria ; 107)

1. Barium. I. Series

ISBN 92 4 157107 1 (NLM Classification: QV 618)
ISSN 0250-863X

©World Health Organization 1990

Publications of the World Health Organization enjoy copyright protection in accordance with the provisions of Protocol 2 of the Universal Copyright Convention. For rights of reproduction or translation of WHO publications, in part or *in toto*, application should be made to the Office of Publications, World Health Organization, Geneva, Switzerland. The World Health Organization welcomes such applications.

The designations employed and the presentation of the material in this publication do not imply the expression of any opinion whatsoever on the part of the Secretariat of the World Health Organization concerning the legal status of any country, territory, city, or area or of its authorities, or concerning the delimitation of its frontiers or boundaries.

The mention of specific companies or of certain manufacturers' products does not imply that they are endorsed or recommended by the World Health Organization in preference to others of a similar nature that are not mentioned. Errors and omissions excepted, the names of proprietary products are distinguished by initial capital letters.

CONTENTS

1. **SUMMARY AND CONCLUSIONS**   13

    1.1 Summary   13
        1.1.1 Identity, natural occurrence, and analytical methods   13
        1.1.2 Production, uses, and sources of exposure   13
        1.1.3 Kinetics and biological monitoring   15
        1.1.4 Effects on experimental animals   17
        1.1.5 Effects on human beings   18
        1.1.6 Effects on organisms in the environment   19
    1.2 Conclusions and recommendations   19

2. **IDENTITY, PHYSICAL AND CHEMICAL PROPERTIES, ANALYTICAL METHODS**   20

    2.1 Identity   20
    2.2 Physical and chemical properties of barium   20
    2.3 Physical and chemical properties of barium compounds   24
    2.4 Analytical sampling   25
        2.4.1 Water   25
        2.4.2 Soils and sediments   25
        2.4.3 Air   26
        2.4.4 Biological materials   26
    2.5 Analytical procedures   26
        2.5.1 Commonly used analytical methods   27
            2.5.1.1 AAS - direct aspiration method   27
            2.5.1.2 AAS - furnace technique   27
            2.5.1.3 AAS - ICP   28
        2.5.2 Analytical methods used for special applications   28
            2.5.2.1 Mass spectrometry   28
            2.5.2.2 X-ray fluorescence spectrometry   28
            2.5.2.3 Neutron activation analysis   29

3. **SOURCES IN THE ENVIRONMENT**   30

    3.1 Natural occurrence   30
    3.2 Man-made sources   31
        3.2.1 Production levels, processes, and uses   31

4.	ENVIRONMENTAL TRANSPORT AND DISTRIBUTION		38
	4.1 Transport and distribution between media		38
		4.1.1 Air	38
		4.1.2 Water	38
		4.1.3 Soil	39
		4.1.4 Vegetation and wildlife	40
		4.1.5 Entry into the food chain	40
	4.2 Biotransformation		40
5.	ENVIRONMENTAL LEVELS AND HUMAN EXPOSURE		41
	5.1 Environmental levels		41
		5.1.1 Air	41
		5.1.2 Water	41
		5.1.2.1 Surface waters	43
		5.1.2.2 Drinking-water	43
		5.1.2.3 Ocean waters	43
		5.1.3 Soil and sediment	44
		5.1.4 Food	44
		5.1.5 Feed	45
		5.1.6 Other products	45
		5.1.7 Nuclear fallout	49
	5.2 General population exposure		50
		5.2.1 Environmental sources, food, drinking-water, and air	50
		5.2.2 Other sources	52
		5.2.3 Subpopulations at special risk	53
	5.3 Occupational exposure during manufacture, formulation, or use		53
6.	KINETICS AND METABOLISM		55
	6.1 Absorption		55
		6.1.1 Inhalation route	55
		6.1.1.1 Laboratory animals	55
		6.1.1.2 Humans	56
		6.1.2 Oral route	57
		6.1.2.1 Laboratory animals	57
		6.1.2.2 Humans	58
		6.1.3 Parenteral administration	58
	6.2 Distribution		58
		6.2.1 Levels in tissues of experimental animals	58
		6.2.2 Levels in human tissue	60

6.3	Elimination and excretion	62
	6.3.1 Laboratory animals	62
	6.3.2 Humans	63
6.4	Metabolism	63
	6.4.1 Laboratory animals	63

7. EFFECTS ON ORGANISMS IN THE ENVIRONMENT 65

7.1	Microorganisms	65
	7.1.1 Viruses	65
	7.1.2 Bacteria	65
	7.1.3 Inhibition of growth	66
	7.1.4 Specific effects	67
7.2	Aquatic organisms	68
	7.2.1 Aquatic plants	68
	7.2.2 Aquatic animals	68
	7.2.3 Effects of marine drilling muds	70
7.3	Bioconcentration	70

8. EFFECTS ON EXPERIMENTAL ANIMALS AND
IN VITRO SYSTEMS 73

8.1	Acute exposure	73
	8.1.1 Oral route	73
	8.1.2 Inhalation route	73
	8.1.3 Parenteral administration	73
	8.1.4 Topical route	75
8.2	Short-term exposures	75
	8.2.1 Inhalation route	75
	8.2.2 Oral route	78
8.3	Long-term exposure	79
	8.3.1 Inhalation route	79
	8.3.2 Oral route	80
8.4	Reproduction, embryotoxicity, and teratogenicity	82
	8.4.1 Reproduction	82
	8.4.2 Embryotoxicity and teratogenicity	82
8.5	Mutagenicity and related end-points	84
8.6	Tumorigenicity and carcinogenicity	84
8.7	Special studies	84
	8.7.1 Effects on the heart	84
	8.7.2 Vascular effects	85
	8.7.3 Electrophysiological effects	86
	8.7.4 Effects on synaptic transmission and catecholamine release	87

	8.7.5 Effects on the immune system	87
	8.7.6 Ocular system	88

9. EFFECTS ON MAN 89

   9.1 General population exposure 89
       9.1.1 Acute toxicity - poisoning incidents 89
       9.1.2 Short-term controlled human studies 91
       9.1.3 Epidemiological studies 92
           9.1.3.1 Cardiovascular disease 92
           9.1.3.2 Other effects 93
   9.2 Occupational exposure 94
       9.2.1 Effects of short- and long-term exposure 94
   9.3 Carcinogenicity of barium chromate 95

10. EVALUATION OF HUMAN HEALTH RISKS AND EFFECTS ON THE ENVIRONMENT 96

   10.1 Evaluation of human health risks 96
       10.1.1 Exposure levels 96
           10.1.1.1 General population 96
           10.1.1.2 Occupational - air exposures 96
           10.1.1.3 Acute exposures 96
       10.1.2 Toxic effects; dose-effect and dose-response relationships 97
       10.1.3 Risk evaluation 98
   10.2 Evaluation of effects on the environment 98

11. RECOMMENDATIONS FOR FURTHER STUDIES 99

12. PREVIOUS EVALUATIONS BY INTERNATIONAL BODIES 100

REFERENCES 101

RESUME ET CONCLUSIONS 122

EVALUATION DES RISQUES POUR LA SANTE HUMAINE ET EFFETS SUR L'ENVIRONNEMENT 131

RECOMMANDATIONS EN VUE D'ETUDES COMPLEMENTAIRES 135

RESUMEN Y CONCLUSIONES 136

EVALUACION DE LOS RIESGOS PARA LA SALUD
HUMANA Y DE LOS EFECTOS SOBRE EL MEDIO
AMBIENTE   144

RECOMENDACIONES PARA ULTERIORES ESTUDIOS   148

WHO TASK GROUP ON ENVIRONMENTAL HEALTH CRITERIA FOR BARIUM

Members

Dr V. Bencko, Department of Hygiene, Institute of Tropical Health, Postgraduate School of Medicine and Pharmacy, Prague, Czechoslovakia

Dr X.C. Ding, Department of Toxicology, Institute of Occupational Health, Shanghai, People's Republic of China[a]

Dr T. Eikmann, Institute for Hygiene and Occupational Medicine, Medical Faculty, Technical University of Rhineland-Westphalia, Aachen, Federal Republic of Germany

Dr J.P. Flesch, Division of Standards Development and Technology Transfer, National Institute for Occupational Safety and Health, Robert A. Taft Laboratories, Cincinnati, Ohio, USA

Ms K. Hughes, Environmental Health Directorate, Department of National Health and Welfare, Tunney's Pasture, Ottawa, Ontario, Canada

Dr F. Izumi, Department of Pharmacology, University of Occupational and Environmental Health, School of Medicine, Fukuoka, Japan

Dr M.L. Tosato, Istituto Superiore di Sanità, Rome, Italy (*Chairperson*)

Secretariat

Dr B.H. Chen, International Programme on Chemical Safety, World Health Organization, Geneva, Switzerland (*Secretary*)

---

[a] Invited but unable to attend.

(Secretariat) contd.

Dr P.G. Jenkins, International Programme on Chemical Safety, World Health Organization, Geneva, Switzerland

Dr T. Ng, Office of Occupational Health, World Health Organization, Geneva, Switzerland

Dr L. Papa, Environmental Criteria and Assessment Office, US Environmental Protection Agency, Cincinnati, Ohio, USA *(Rapporteur)*

NOTE TO READERS OF THE CRITERIA MONOGRAPHS

Every effort has been made to present information in the criteria monographs as accurately as possible without unduly delaying their publication. In the interest of all users of the environmental health criteria monographs, readers are kindly requested to communicate any errors that may have occurred to the Manager of the International Programme on Chemical Safety, World Health Organization, Geneva, Switzerland, in order that they may be included in corrigenda, which will appear in subsequent volumes.

* * *

A detailed data profile and a legal file can be obtained from the International Register of Potentially Toxic Chemicals, Palais des Nations, 1211 Geneva 10, Switzerland (Telephone No. 7988400 or 7985850).

ENVIRONMENTAL HEALTH CRITERIA FOR BARIUM

A WHO Task Group on Environmental Health Criteria for Barium met in Geneva from 20 to 24 November 1989. Dr M. Mercier, Manager, IPCS, opened the meeting and welcomed the participants on behalf of the heads of the three IPCS cooperating organizations (UNEP/ILO/WHO). The Task Group reviewed and revised the draft criteria monograph and made an evaluation of the risks for human health and the environment from exposure to barium.

The first draft of this monograph was prepared by Dr L. PAPA of the US Environmental Protection Agency. The second draft was also prepared by Dr L. Papa, incorporating comments received following the circulation of the first draft to the IPCS Contact Points for Environmental Health Criteria documents. Dr B.H. Chen and Dr P.G. Jenkins, both members of the IPCS Central Unit, were responsible for the overall scientific content and editing, respectively.

The efforts of all who helped in the preparation and finalization of the document are gratefully acknowledged.

ABBREVIATIONS

AAS   Atomic absorption spectrophotometry

BUN   Blood urea nitrogen

CNS   Central nervous system

ECG   Electrocardiogram

IARC International Agency for Research on Cancer

ip   Intraperitoneal

iv   Intravenous

LLD   Lowest lethal dose

PNS   Peripheral nervous system

sc   Subcutaneous

1. SUMMARY AND CONCLUSIONS

1.1 Summary

1.1.1 Identity, natural occurrence, and analytical methods

Barium is one of the alkaline earth metals, having a relative atomic mass of 137.34 and an atomic number of 56. It has seven naturally occurring stable isotopes, of which ^{138}Ba is the most abundant. Barium is a yellowish-white soft metal that is strongly electropositive. It combines with ammonia, water, oxygen, hydrogen, halogens, and sulfur, energy being released by these reactions. It also reacts strongly with metals to form metal alloys. In nature barium occurs only in a combined state, the principal mineral forms being barite (barium sulfate) and witherite (barium carbonate). Barium is also present in small quantities in igneous rocks and in feldspar and micas. It may be found as a natural component of fossil fuel and is present in air, water, and soil.

Certain barium compounds, such as acetate, nitrate, and chloride are relatively water soluble, whereas the fluoride, carbonate, oxalate, chromate, phosphate, and sulfate salts have very low solubility. With the exception of barium sulfate, the water solubility of the barium salts increases with decreasing pH.

Sampling of barium in aqueous and gaseous media is conducted in the same way as it is for any other material. Sediments, sludge, and soil samples are oven-dried or sintered. The samples are then extracted in 1% HCl for analysis of trace elements, including barium. Biological samples are frozen or lyophilized and are prepared for barium analysis using dry-washing procedures.

Atomic absorption and flame and plasma emission spectrometry are the most commonly employed analytical methods. Neutron activation, isotope dilution mass spectrometry, and X-ray fluorescence are also used.

1.1.2 Production, uses, and sources of exposure

Barite ore is the raw material from which nearly all other barium compounds are derived. World production of barite in 1985 was estimated to be 5.7 million tonnes. Barium and its compounds are used in diverse industrial products ranging from ceramics to lubricants. It is used in the manufacture of alloys, as a loader for paper, soap, rubber, and linoleum, in the manufacture of valves, and as an extinguisher for radium, uranium, and plutonium fires.

Anthropogenic sources of barium are primarily industrial. Emissions may result from mining, refining, or processing of barium minerals and manufacture of barium products. Barium is also discharged in waste water from metallurgical and industrial processes. Deposition on soil may result from man's activities, including the disposal of fly ash and primary and secondary sludge in landfill. It was estimated that in 1976, mining and processing of barite ore in the USA released approximately 3200 tonnes of particulates into the air, and fugitive dusts from the use of barite in oil drilling and oil-related industries accounted for approximately 100 tonnes of particulates. In 1972, the barium chemical industry in the USA released an estimated 1200 tonnes of particulates into the atmosphere.

Environmental transport of barium occurs through the air, water, and soil. Atmospheric barium consists of particulates whose transport is regulated by normal atmospheric and meteorological circumstances. Transport of barium in water is subject to interaction with other ions, including sulfate, which regulates and limits barium concentration. Little information is available regarding the aqueous transformations and transport of barium.

Exposure to barium can occur through air, water, or food. The levels of barium in the air are not well documented. In the USA, the usual concentration is estimated to be 0.05 $\mu g/m^3$ or less. No distinct correlation has been observed between ambient levels of barium in the air and the extent of industrialization, although higher concentrations occur around smelters.

The presence of barium in sea water, river water, and well-water has been documented, and it is also found in sediments and natural waters in contact with sedimentary rocks. Barium is present in almost all surface waters at concentrations up to 15 000 μg/litre and contributes to the hardness of the water. The barium concentration in wells depends on the content of leachable barium in rocks. Drinking-water contains 10-1000 µg/litre, although water in certain regions of the USA has been shown to have concentrations in excess of 10 000 µg/litre. Municipal water supplies depend upon the quality of surface and ground water and, depending on the hardness, contain a wide range of barium concentration. Studies from USA show levels in drinking-water ranging from 1-20 µg/litre. Based on this information and assuming a consumption rate of 2 litres per day, the daily intake would be 2-40 µg barium.

Several studies have estimated a daily dietary intake range of 300-1770 µg with large variations. Humans seldom eat plants in which barium is present in significant amounts or the part of the plant in which the barium accumulates. The Brazil nut tree is an exception, reported concentrations being 1500-3000 µg/g. Tomatoes and soy bean are also known to concentrate soil barium, the bioconcentration factor ranging from 2 to 20.

In general, barium does not accumulate in common plants in sufficient quantities to be toxic to animals. However, it has been suggested that the large quantities of barium (as high as 1260 mg/kg) accumulated in legumes, alfalfa, and soybeans could cause problems in domestic cattle.

The barium content of dry tobacco leaves averages 105 mg/kg, most of which is likely to remain in the ash during burning. No values for barium concentrations in tobacco smoke have been reported.

Another source of barium exposure is nuclear fallout. However, with the establishment of atmospheric test ban treaties, the quantity of radioactive barium in the environment has decreased.

1.1.3   *Kinetics and biological monitoring*

The average person (70 kg) contains approximately 22 mg of barium, most of which (91%) is localized in the bone. Trace quantities are found in various tissues such as the aorta, brain, heart, kidney, spleen, pancreas, and lung. Total barium in human beings tends to increase with age. The levels in the body depend on the geographical location of the individual. Barium has also been found in

Summary and Conclusions

all samples of stillborn babies, suggesting that it can cross the placenta.

It is difficult to assess the uptake of ingested barium because a number of factors affect absorption. For instance, the presence of sulfate in food results in the precipitation of barium sulfate. Studies on experimental animals and limited human data indicate that soluble barium is absorbed through the intestine to the extent of < 10% in adults but more in the young. Uptake occurs rapidly in the salivary and adrenal glands, heart, kidney, mucosal tissue and blood vessels, and finally in the skeleton. Like calcium, barium accumulates in bone. It is deposited preferentially in the most active areas of bone growth, primarily at the periosteal surfaces. Other factors important in absorption and deposition include age and dietary restriction. Older rats exhibit decreased absorption and bone concentrations of barium. Fasting elicits an increase in barium absorption.

Inhaled barium can be absorbed through the lung or directly from the nasal membrane into the bloodstream. In rats, exposure results in deposition in the bones, but continued exposure results in decreased deposition both in the bones and the lungs. Insoluble compounds, such as barium sulfate, accumulate in the lungs and are cleared slowly by ciliary action.

Barium is eliminated in the urine and in the faeces, the rates varying with the route of administration. Within 24 h, approximately 20% of a barium dose, injected into humans, was eliminated in the faeces and approximately 5% in the urine. Plasma barium is almost entirely cleared from the bloodstream within 24 h. The elimination of ingested barium in both human beings and animals occurs principally in the faeces rather than in the urine. Following inhalation exposure, there is a slow elimination of barium from bone and, thus, from the whole body. An estimate of the biological half-life for barium in the rat is 90-120 days. For adequate biological monitoring of human exposure, the elimination of barium in urine as well as in faeces should be monitored.

1.1.4 Effects on experimental animals

In the rat, oral LD_{50} values of 118, 250, and 355 were measured for barium chloride, fluoride, and nitrate, respectively. The acute effects of barium ingestion include salivation, nausea, diarrhoea, tachycardia, hypokalaemia, twitching, flaccid paralysis of skeletal muscle, respiratory muscle paralysis, and ventricular fibrillation. Respiratory muscle paralysis and ventricular fibrillation may lead to death. Various studies have demonstrated the detrimental effect of barium upon ventricular automaticity and pacemaker current in the heart. Intravenous barium injections to anaesthetized dogs indicated that these acute effects were due to prompt and substantial hypokalaemia and could be prevented or reversed by potassium administration.

Barium causes mild skin and severe eye irritation in rabbits.

When rats ingested tap water containing up to 250 mg barium/litre for 13 weeks, no signs of toxicity were observed, although some groups showed a decrease in the relative weight of the adrenals.

Rats given 10 or 100 mg barium/litre in their drinking-water for 16 months experienced hypertension, but a level of 1 mg/litre did not induce any blood pressure changes. Analysis of myocardial function at 16 months (100 mg barium/litre) revealed significantly altered cardiac contractility and excitability, myocardial metabolic disturbances, and hypersensitivity of the cardiovascular system to sodium pentobarbital.

Oral or inhalation administration of barium carbonate in rats resulted in adverse reproductive effects. In addition, the death rate was higher for the newborn offspring of barium-treated dams. There is limited evidence of teratogenicity of barium, but no conclusive evidence of carcinogenicity is available.

Barium possesses chemical and physiological properties that allow it to compete with and replace calcium in processes mediated normally by calcium, particularly those relating to the release of adrenal catecholamines and neurotransmitters, such as acetylcholine and noradrenaline.

Limited information is available regarding the immunological effects of barium in animals.

1.1.5 Effects on human beings

Several cases of poisoning due to the ingestion of barium compounds have been reported. Barium doses as low as 0.2-0.5 mg/kg body weight, generally resulting from the ingestion of barium chloride or carbonate, have been found to lead to toxic effects in adult humans. Clinical features of barium poisoning include acute gastroenteritis, loss of deep reflexes with onset of muscular paralysis, and progressive muscular paralysis. The muscular paralysis appears to be related to severe hypokalaemia. In most reported cases, rapid and uneventful recovery occurred after treatment with infused potassium salts (carbonate or lactate) and/or oral administration of sodium sulfate.

Limited epidemiological studies have been conducted to investigate the possible relationship between barium concentrations in drinking-water and cardiovascular mortality, but the results have been inconsistent and inconclusive.

No increase in the incidence of elevated blood pressure, stroke, or heart and kidney disease was observed in a population exposed to high concentrations of barium in drinking-water when compared to a similar group exposed to lower levels. In a short-term human volunteer study, no effects on blood pressure were induced by the consumption of barium in drinking-water.

An increase in the incidence of hypertension was reported among workers exposed to barium, compared with non-exposed workers. Baritosis has been observed in individuals occupationally exposed to barium compounds. A study group consisting of barium-exposed workers and people residing near a landfill site containing barium was found to have an increased prevalence of musculoskeletal symptoms, gastrointestinal surgery, skin problems, and respiratory symptoms.

No conclusive association was found between the level of barium in drinking-water and the incidence of congenital malformations. There is no evidence that barium is carcinogenic.

1.1.6 Effects on organisms in the environment

Barium directly affects the physico-chemical properties as well as the infectivity of several viruses and their ability to multiply. It also affects the development of germinating bacterial spores and has a variety of specific effects on different microorganisms, including the inhibition of cellular processes.

Little information is available on the effects of barium on aquatic organisms. There were no effects on survival in fish following exposure for 30 days. However, in a 21-day study, impairment of reproduction and reduction in growth were observed in daphnids at a dose of 5.8 mg barium/litre. No evidence has been found to indicate that barite is toxic to marine animals. However, exposure to barite in large amounts could adversely affect colonization by benthic animals.

Marine plants, as well as invertebrates, may actively accumulate barium from sea water.

1.2 Conclusions and recommendations

Barium, at concentrations normally found in our environment, does not pose any significant risk for the general population. However, for specific subpopulations and under conditions of high barium exposure, the potential for adverse health effects should be taken into account.

Few data are available for evaluating the risk to the environment posed by barium. However, based on the available information on the toxic effects of barium in daphnids, it appears that barium may represent a risk to populations of some aquatic organisms.

There is a need for epidemiological studies, for research on bioavailability and cardiovascular and immunological toxicity, and for additional information on chronic aquatic toxicity. In order to establish better protection measures, more data on exposures in the workplace and the use of biomarkers are necessary.

2. IDENTITY, PHYSICAL AND CHEMICAL PROPERTIES, ANALYTICAL METHODS

2.1 Identity

Barium is a member of the alkaline earth metals in Group IIA of the periodic table, along with beryllium, magnesium, calcium, strontium, and radium. The symbol for the element is Ba. Barium has an atomic number of 56 and a relative atomic mass of 137.34. The CAS registry and RTECS registry numbers for barium are 7440-39-3 and CQ8370000, respectively. Metallic barium is obtained by reducing barium oxide with aluminum or silicon in a vacuum at high temperature.

Twenty-five barium isotopes have been identified (CRC, 1988). There are seven naturally occurring stable isotopes with mass numbers of 130, 132, 134, 135, 136, 137, and 138, ^{138}Ba being the most abundant (Lederer et al., 1967). The others are unstable isotopes with half-lives ranging from 12.8 days for ^{140}Ba to 12 seconds for ^{143}Ba (CRC, 1988). Two of these isotopes, ^{131}Ba and ^{139}Ba, are used in research as radioactive tracers. A list of common barium compounds with their formulae and CAS registry numbers is presented in Table 1.

2.2 Physical and chemical properties of barium

Important physical and chemical properties of barium relevant to exposure assessment and effects are shown in Table 2. It is a silver-white, soft metal, relatively volatile and readily distilled (Goodenough & Stenger, 1973). Powdered barium is pyrophoric and very dangerous to handle in the presence of air or other oxidizing gases (Quagliano, 1959). As might be expected from its high electrode potential (-2.912 V), barium is extremely reactive and the free energy of formation of its compounds is very high. Therefore it does not exist in nature in the elemental state but occurs as the divalent cation, Ba^{2+}, in combination with other elements. Barium reacts readily with halogens, oxygen, and sulfur to form halides, oxide, and sulfide. It also reacts with nitrogen and hydrogen at

Table 1. Common barium compounds[a]

Substance	Formula	CAS No.	RTECS No.
Aluminium barium titanium oxide	Not given	52869-91-7	BD 0345400
Barium acetate	$Ba(C_2H_3O_2)_2 \cdot H_2O$	543-80-6	AF 4550000
Barium azide	$Ba(N_3)_2$	18810-58-7	CQ 8500000
Barium bromate	$Ba(BrO_3)_2 \cdot H_2O$	13967-90-3	EF 8715000
Barium cadmium laurate	$(C_{12}H_{24}O_2)_4 \cdot Ba \cdot Cd$	Not given	OE 9805000
Barium cadmium stearate	$(C_{18}H_{36}O_2)_4 \cdot Ba \cdot Cd$	1191-79-3	WI 2830000
Barium calcium titanium oxide	Not given	52869-93-9	CQ 8580000
Barium carbonate	$BaCO_3$	513-77-9	CQ 8600000
Barium chlorate	$Ba(ClO_3)_2 \cdot H_2O$	13477-00-4	FN 9770000
Barium chloride	$BaCl_2$	10361-37-2	CQ 8950000
Barium chloride, dihydrate	$BaCl_2 \cdot 2H_2O$	10326-27-9	CQ 8751000
Barium chromate (VI)	$BaCrO_4$	10294-40-3	CQ 8760000
Barium cyanide	$Ba(CN)_2$	542-62-1	CQ 8785000
Barium fluoborate	$Ba(BF_4)_2$	13862-62-9	CQ 8925000
Barium fluoride	BaF_2	7787-32-8	CQ 9100000

Identity, Physical and Chemical Properties, Analytical Methods

Table 1 (contd).

Substance	Formula	CAS No.	RTECS No.
Barium hypochlorite	$Ba(ClO_2)_2$	13477-10-6	NH 3480000
Barium iron oxide	$BaFe_{12}O_{19}$	12047-11-9	CQ 9520800
Barium nitrate	$Ba(NO_3)_2$	10022-31-8	CQ 9625000
Barium oxide	BaO	1304-28-5	CQ 9800000
Barium perchlorate	$Ba(ClO_4)_2 \cdot 4H_2O$	13465-95-7	SC 7550000
Barium permanganate	$Ba(MnO_4)_2$	7787-36-2	SD 6405000
Barium peroxide	BaO_2	1304-29-6	CR 0175000
Barium silicofluoride	$BaSiF_6$	17125-80-3	CR 0525000
Barium sulfate	$BaSO_4$	7727-43-7	CR 0600000
Barium sulfide	BaS	50864-67-0	CR 0270000
Barium sulfide, mixture with sulfur	Not given	8077-30-3	CR 0660000
Barium sulfonates	Not given	Not given	CR 0700000
Barium zirconium (IV) oxide	$BaZr_4O_4$	12009-21-1	CR 0875000

[a] Source: RTECS (1985).

Table 2. Physical and chemical properties of barium[a]

Atomic number	56
Relative atomic mass	137.34
Physical state	solid metal
Colour	yellowish-white
Melting point	725 °C
Boiling point	1640 °C
Solubility in water	reacts with release of H_2
Solubility in alcohol	soluble (decomposes)
Solubility in benzene	insoluble
Relative density (at 20 °C)	3.51
Extremely reactive with	water, ammonia, halogens, oxygen most acids
Electrode potential ($E°(aq)Ba^{2+}/Ba$) (at 25 °C, 1 atm.)	-2.912 volts
Electronegativity	1.02
Flame coloration test	green

[a] Source: Weast (1983), Windholz (1983).

higher temperatures to form the nitride and hydride, and it reacts vigorously with water displacing hydrogen to form the hydroxide. Treatment of barium hydroxide with hydrogen peroxide at low temperatures forms barium peroxide, which can also be formed by direct combination of oxygen with barium oxide or the metal. Barium exhibits little tendency to form complexes; the amines formed with NH_3 are unstable and the *beta*-diketons and alcoholates are not well characterized.

Barium attacks most metals with the formation of alloys; iron is the most resistant to alloy formation. Barium forms alloys and intermetallic compounds with lead, potassium, platinum, magnesium, silicon, zinc, aluminium, and mercury (Hansen, 1958). Metallic barium reduces the oxides, halides, and sulfides of most of the less reactive metals, thereby producing the corresponding metal.

2.3 Physical and chemical properties of barium compounds

Barium compounds exhibit close relationships with the compounds of calcium and strontium, which are also alkaline earth metals. The physical and chemical properties of various barium compounds are listed in Table 3. Barium acetate, nitrate, and chloride are quite soluble, whereas the arsenate, carbonate, oxalate, chromate, fluoride, sulfate, and phosphate salts are very poorly soluble. All barium salts, except for barium sulfate, become increasingly soluble as the pH decreases. These salts dissolve partially in carbonic acid and completely in hydrochloric or nitric acids. Strong sulfuric acid is required to dissolve barium sulfate.

Table 3. Physical and chemical properties of various barium compounds[a]

Compound	Relative molecular mass	Relative density	Solubility in water[b]	Melting point[c] (°C)	Boiling point (°C)
Barium acetate	255.45	2.468	58.80	-	-
Barium arsenate	689.83	5.10	0.55	1605	-
Barium carbonate	197.37	4.43	0.02	1790 (90)	-
Barium chloride	208.25	3.856	375 (26)	962	1560
Barium chromate	253.32	4.498	0.0034 (16)	-	-
Barium fluoride	175.34	4.89	1.2 (25)	1375	2137
Barium hydroxide·8H_2O	315.47	2.18	56 (15)	78	78 (-8H_2O)
Barium nitrate	261.38	3.24	87	592	[d]
Barium oxalate	225.35	2.658	0.093 (18)	400[d]	-
Barium oxide	153.36	5.72	34.8	1918	≈2000
Barium phosphate, dibasic	233.5	4.165	0.1-0.2	410 (710)[d]	-
Barium triphosphate	601.93	4.10	insoluble	-	-
Barium sulfate	233.4	4.5	0.002	1580	-

[a] CRC (1988).
[b] in g/litre at 20 °C; where the solubility was not measured at 20 °C, the temperature used is shown in parentheses.
[c] at 760 mmHg; where the pressure was otherwise, it is given in parentheses.
[d] decomposes.

In aqueous solution, the barium ion can combine with organic chelating agents. Owing to its similarity to calcium in its chemical properties and because it lies below calcium in the periodic table, barium is thought to interact with biochemical pathways involving calcium ion-binding by competing for binding sites of chelation (Sillen & Martell, 1964). Barium may also bind with organic ligands to form biological complexes.

2.4 Analytical sampling

Barium does not require sampling or handling procedures different from those used in general analytical practice. The greatest sources of sampling error in environmental studies are the variations in the material being sampled. Sampling procedures must not only take into account the physical and chemical properties of the specific barium compound but must also accurately reflect variations in the media (water, air, and soil).

2.4.1 Water

The US EPA (1979a) recommended the following procedure for sampling and preserving metals in aqueous solution. A minimum of 200 ml is collected in an analytically clean container, preferably made of polyethylene, with a polypropylene cap (no liner). For the determination of dissolved constituents (i.e. barium), the sample must be filtered through a membrane filter (0.45 μm) preferably on-site. The suspended constituents retained by the membrane filter are saved if total barium analysis is required. The filtered sample may be initially preserved by icing. However, as soon as possible, the sample must be acidified to a pH <2 with nitric acid (normally 3 ml 1:1 nitric acid per litre is sufficient). A maximum holding time of 6 months is recommended, although the length of time will also depend on the type of sample used.

2.4.2 Soils and sediments

Samples of soils, sediments, and sludge are oven-dried and stored in polyethylene containers. The samples are extracted in 1% hydrochloric acid for analysis of trace elements including barium (Fortescue et al., 1976). Samples of benthic intertidal sediments from sandy beaches can be stored in clean polyethylene bottles and frozen (-15 °C) (Chow et al., 1978). Benthic sediments are collected with a non-contaminating box-core device, with only the top 1 cm of the core being saved.

2.4.3 Air

Barium is sampled in the same way as other compounds in air. A known volume of air is drawn through a cellulose filter to collect the compound in the particulate fraction (NIOSH, 1977). Samples collected on the filters are leached into hot water, filtered, and dried.

2.4.4 Biological materials

Biological tissues such as hair, blood, and placenta are kept frozen or lyophilized before analysing for barium (Creason et al., 1976). Dry-washing procedures are used to prepare the samples for barium analysis. Research at the National Bureau of Standards, Washington, DC, indicated that bovine liver samples, lyophilized and ground, showed no change in composition after prolonged storage at room temperature (Becker, 1976). Similar procedures were used for orchard plant leaves. Samples carefully dried and lyophilized can be adequately stored at room temperature for several years with no significant changes in trace metal composition (Becker, 1976).

2.5 Analytical procedures

In general, analytical procedures measure total barium ion present rather than specific barium compounds.

Analysis for soluble barium in aqueous solutions requires consideration of contaminating substances that may interfere with the assay. Certain contaminants can affect absorption as well as emission spectra. Maruta et al. (1972) observed that the presence of aluminum depressed the barium signal and that the addition of alkali compounds (except caesium) suppressed barium ionization. Magill & Svehla (1974) also noted that several anions and cations interfered with the analysis of barium.

Separation of barium from interfering components is achieved by ion-exchange chromatography. Akiyama & Tomita (1973) employed a chromium phosphate ion exchanger. Other workers have used Dowex 50 ion-exchange resin, with various degrees of cross linking (Dybczynski, 1972; Wolgemuth & Broecker, 1970; Bacon & Edmond, 1972; Pierce & Brown, 1977). Elution is carried out with hydrochloric acid. Pierce & Brown (1977) used a chelating agent, ethylenediamine tetraacetic acid (EDTA), to elute barium from the Dowex 50 column in a semi-automated procedure. Quantification of low concentrations of barium using chemical methods (wet, gravimetric) is at present seldom attempted. Owing to the high ionization properties of barium and spectral interference from calcium emissions, the use of instrumental methods for analysing barium is often difficult.

2.5.1 Commonly used analytical methods

Atomic absorption spectrophotometry (AAS) is a readily available and widely used analytical technique for determining several metals in solution from a variety of samples. The US EPA (1974, 1979a) recommends two AAS methods for barium, the direct aspiration method and the furnace technique.

2.5.1.1 AAS - Direct aspiration method

The optimal concentration range for determining barium by the AAS direct aspiration method, using a wavelength of 553.6 nm, is 1-20 mg/litre, with a sensitivity of 0.4 mg/litre and a detection limit of 0.03 mg/litre (US EPA, 1979a). An AAS direct aspiration method for the determination of water-soluble barium components in air has been described by NIOSH (1977). The air sample is drawn through a cellulose membrane filter on which the analyte is collected. The working range of the method was estimated to be 0.15-1.3 mg/m^3, with a sensitivity of 0.0004 mg/m^3.

2.5.1.2 AAS - Furnace technique

For concentrations of barium <0.2 mg/litre, the furnace technique is recommended. The optimal concentration range for barium determination by the furnace technique is 10-200 µg/litre, the detection limit being 2 µg/litre. A detection limit of 0.5 ng/ml using a 20 µl sample was also reported for this method (Slavin, 1984). The Association of Official Analytical Chemists (AOAC, 1984) used emission spectrography for measuring barium concentrations in plant tissue. The coefficient of variation for barium analysis was between 7 and 15%, depending on the type of plant tissue analysed. The analysis of barium in drinking-water was performed by Pierce & Brown (1977) using this method; they reported a detection limit and sensitivity for barium of 3.0 and 10.0 µg/litre, respectively.

2.5.1.3 AAS - ICP

In recent years, emission spectrometry employing an inductively coupled plasma (ICP) source has been used routinely (Garbarino & Taylor, 1979). Detection limits of ≤ 0.1 ng/ml have been reported (Fassel & Kniseley, 1974), with less of the chemical or ionization interference typically seen with other emission spectroscopic systems. Optical emission methods, however, are expensive when used for a single element analysis, but this problem is largely offset when several elements are analysed simultaneously.

2.5.2 *Analytical methods used for special applications*

2.5.2.1 *Mass spectrometry*

Because of expense and low sample throughput, mass spectrometry is not a commonly used procedure for the analysis of barium or other elements. However, aqueous barium samples, purified by ion exchange, are particularly amenable to this procedure (Bacon & Edmond, 1972). Peaks for ^{135}Ba and ^{138}Ba can be scanned and replicate analyses can be performed with a coefficient of variation of 0.17%. Isotope dilution mass spectrometry is an extremely valuable reference method. Several investigators have indicated that the isotope dilution mass spectrometric method circumvents the need for large samples and tedious purification procedures. Internal standardization provides a high degree of precision, element selectivity, and sensitivity (Chow & Patterson, 1966; Wolgemuth & Broecker, 1970; Bernat et al., 1972).

2.5.2.2 *X-ray fluorescence spectrometry*

This technique has been used to measure barium concentrations in human tissue (Forssen & Erametsa, 1974) and in river sediments (Tsai et al., 1978). The coefficient of variation of this method was 5.6% when river sediments were analysed (Tsai et al., 1978).

2.5.2.3 *Neutron activation analysis*

Neutron activation can be used for multi-element analysis. This technique has been used to determine barium in sludge (Nadkarni & Morrison, 1974), in marine sediments (Chow et al., 1978), and biological tissues (Heffron et al., 1977). The correlation coefficient of the data when compared with isotope dilution methods is 0.923, and the limit of detection is 1 µg (Reeves, 1986).

3. SOURCES IN THE ENVIRONMENT

3.1 Natural occurrence

Barium is a relatively abundant element found combined with other elements in soils, rocks, and minerals. It ranks seventh in abundance among the minor elements and sixteenth among the non-gaseous elements in the earth's crust (Schroeder, 1970), and constitutes about 0.04% of the earth's crust (Reeves, 1979). Barium also occurs as gangue in lead and zinc ore deposits. The terrestrial abundance of barium has been estimated at 250 g/tonne, and its occurrence in sea water is 0.006 g/tonne (Considine, 1976).

The two most prevalent naturally occurring compounds of barium are barite (barium sulfate) and witherite (barium carbonate). Barite crystallizes in the orthorhombic system. It occurs in beds or masses in limestone, dolomite, shales, and other sedimentary formations; as residual nodules resulting from the weathering of barite-bearing dolomite or limestone; and as gangue in beds together with fluorspar, metallic sulfides, and other minerals.

Witherite crystallizes in the orthorhombic system. It is found in veins and is often associated with galena (lead sulfide), as at Alston Moor, Cumberland, England. It is also found associated with barite at Freiberg, Saxony, German Democratic Republic, and at Lexington, Kentucky, USA.

Barium occurs in coal at concentrations up to 3000 mg/kg (Bowen, 1966). It also occurs in fuel oils, the barium content varying with the petroleum source.

Barium is ubiquitous in soils, being found at concentrations ranging from 100-3000 μg/g (Schroeder, 1970; Robinson et al., 1950). Brooks (1978) estimated an average soil concentration of 500 mg/kg. Due to its abundance in soils, barium may be present in the air in areas with high natural dust levels.

Barium can be transported into ground-water aquifers through the leaching and eroding of barium from sedimentary rocks. The level of barium present in the ground water is related to the hardness of the water, since barium is always present with calcium (Kopp & Kroner, 1968). Cartwright et al. (1978) reported that the high barium levels in ground water in Illinois, USA, were derived from the sandstone formation of the Cambrian-Ordovician aquifer. The highest concentrations occurred in fine-grained and older sediments. Barium was found in 94% of the surface waters examined, the concentrations range being 2-340 µg/litre (Kopp & Kroner, 1967).

Barium in surface waters is ultimately transported into the oceans where it combines with the sulfate ion present in salt water to form barium sulfate. Barium in the ocean is in a steady state; the amount entering from rivers is balanced by the amount falling to the bottom as particles to form a permanent part of the sediment on the ocean floor (Wolgemuth & Brocker, 1970). Barium concentrations in sea water of 6 µg/litre and in fresh water of 7-15 000 µg/litre (an average of 50 µg/litre) have been reported (Reeves, 1986).

3.2 Man-made sources

3.2.1 Production levels, processes, and uses

Barite ore is the raw material from which nearly all other barium compounds are derived. World production of barite in 1985 was estimated to be approximately 5.7 million tonnes. The major world producers of barite are China, the United States, USSR, India, Mexico, Morocco, Ireland, Federal Republic of Germany, and Thailand. Other producers are Canada, France, Spain, Czechoslovakia, and England (Vagt, 1985).

China, as the world's leading producer, accounted for about 1.0 million tonnes or 17% of world output in 1984. The USA, the second largest producer, accounted for 0.70 million tonnes in 1984 and also imported 1.6 million tonnes. Canada produced approximately 64 000 tonnes and consumed around 78 000 tonnes in 1984 (Vagt, 1985).

Emissions of barium into the air from mining, refining, and processing barium ore can occur during loading and unloading, stock-piling, materials handling, and grinding and refining of the ore. According to emission factors determined by Davis (1972), mining and processing of barite ore released an estimated 3200 tonnes of particulates into the air in 1976 in the USA (US Bureau of Mines, 1976). Emission into water may occur during the purification of barite ore and subsequent discharge of the industrial water to the environment.

Fossil fuel combustion may also release barium into the air. Pierson et al. (1981) found that >90% of the barium additive in diesel fuels is emitted in vehicle exhaust, where it is totally in the form of barium sulfate.

Coal-fired power plants emit barium into the atmosphere via ash. Some barium escapes into the atmosphere as fly ash (Cuffe & Gerstle, 1967), while the rest is generally disposed of in landfill. Barium in coal ash ranges from 100-5000 mg/kg (Miner, 1969). Hildebrand et al. (1976) reported the presence of barium at a concentration of 0.02 mg/litre in the effluent from a coal conversion plant.

In the USA, the barium chemical industries released an estimated 1200 tonnes of particulates into the atmosphere in 1972 (Davis, 1972; Rezink & Toy, 1978). Waste water from barium chemical production processes is another potential source of barium emission.

Although most fugitive dust emissions and process effluents are reduced by control technologies, an area of concern is the emission of soluble barium to the atmosphere from dryers and calciners. Baghouses can reduce the uncontrolled emission factor (up to 10 g/kg final product) to 0.25 g/kg (Rezink & Toy, 1978). The release of soluble barium into the atmosphere around these plants was estimated at 56 tonnes for 1972 (Rezink & Toy, 1978), but it has decreased as barium chemical production has declined. The plastics industry is a relatively important source of barium emission to the atmosphere. It utilizes barium as a stabilizer to prevent discoloration during processing.

Another source of barium emission is the manufacture of glass. Emissions of barium-containing particulates with an average size of 1 μm have been reported by various authors (Stockham, 1971; Davis, 1972). Davis (1972) estimated an emission of 1 kg/1000 kg of barium used in the glass industry. In a study of glass furnace emissions, Stockham (1971) found negligible emissions of barium in the formation of flint glass but a 1-10% emission level of the particulates in the effluent of amber glass manufacturing.

The detonation of nuclear devices in the atmosphere is a source of atmospheric radioactive barium. The radioactive isotopes ^{140}Ba and ^{143}Ba are products of the decay chains from thermal-neutron fission of ^{235}U. Among the isotopes of barium, ^{140}Ba has the longest half-life (12.8 days) and contributes 10% of the total fission products at 10 days after nuclear fission. At 60 days, however, its contribution falls to 2% of total activity (French, 1963). The concentration of barium particles in the atmosphere due to this source, in terms of actual weight, is immeasurably small. Due to the short half-life and low concentrations of barium radionuclides, this source is not considered a significant source of barium in the environment.

Barium is used extensively by man and is an essential component of a vast number of manufacturing processes, some of which are identified in Table 4. It is used in the manufacture of alloys, as a loader for paper, soap, rubber, and linoleum, in the manufacture of valves, and in the production of lights and green flares. Barium is also used in cement where concrete is exposed to salt water, in the radio industry to capture the last traces of gases in vacuum tubes, in the ceramic and glass industries, as an insecticide and rodenticide, and as an extinguisher for radium, uranium, and plutonium fires (Browning, 1969).

Barite is a valuable industrial mineral because of its high specific gravity, low abrasiveness, chemical stability, and lack of magnetic effects. Its main use is as a weighting agent for oil- and gas-well drilling muds required to counteract high pressures confined by the substrata. The oil- and gas-well drilling industries used 90% of the 2.24 million tonnes of barite consumed in the USA in 1976 (US Bureau of Mines, 1976). In the same year, unloading and handling this material released an estimated 112 tonnes of particulates into the atmosphere (Davis, 1972; US Bureau of Mines, 1976).

Table 4. Main uses of some barium compounds[a]

Barium compound	Uses
Acetate	Catalyst for organic reactions; textile mordant; oil and grease lubricator; paint and varnish driers
Aluminate	In ceramics; in water treatment
Azide	In high explosives
Bromate	Analytical reagent; oxidizing agent; corrosion inhibitor in low carbon steel; in the preparation of rare earth bromates
Bromide	In the manufacture of other bromides; in photographic compounds; in the preparation of phosphors
Carbonate	In the treatment of brines in chlorinealkali cells to remove sulfates; as a rodenticide; in ceramic flux, optical glass, case-hardening baths, ferrites, radiation-resistant glass for colour television tubes; in manufacturing paper
Chlorate	In pyrotechnics (green fire); as textile mordant; in the manufacture of other chlorates and of explosives and matches
Chloride	In the manufacture of pigments, colour lakes, glass; as a mordant for acid dyes; in pesticides, lube oil additives, boiler compounds, and aluminum refining; as a flux in the manufacture of magnesium metal; in leather tanner and finisher, in photographic paper and textiles
Chromate	In safety matches; as a pigment in paints; in ceramics; in fuses; in pyrotechnics; in metal primers; in ignition control devices
Citrate	As a stabilizer for latex paints
Cyanide	In metallurgy and electroplating
Cyanoplatinite	In X-ray screens
Diphenylamine sulfonate	As an indicator in oxidation-reduction titrations
Ethylsulfate	In organic preparations
Fluoride	In ceramics; in the manufacture of other fluorides; in crystals for spectroscopy; in electronics; in dry-film lubricants; in embalming; in glass manufacture; manufacture of carbon brushes for DC motors and generators
Fluorosilicate	In ceramics; in insecticidal compositions; in the preparation of silicon tetrafluoride
Hydroxide, monohydrate	In the manufacture of oil and grease additives; in barium soaps and chemicals; in the refinishing of beet sugar and animal and vegetable oils; as an alkalizing agent in water softening; as a sulfate removal agent in the treatment of water and brine; in boiler scale removal; as a depilatory agent; as a catalyst in the manufacture of phenol-formaldehyde resins; as insecticide and fungicide; as a sulfate-controlling agent in ceramics; as a purifying agent for caustic soda; as a steel carbonizing agent; in glass; synthetic rubber vulcanization; as a corrosion inhibitor; in drilling fluids, lubricants

Table 4 (contd).

Barium compound	Uses
Hydroxide, octahydrate and pentahydrate	In organic preparations; in barium salts; in analytical chemistry (and uses described for the monohydrate)
Hypophosphite	In medicine and nickel plating
Iodide	In the preparation of other iodides
Manganate (VI)	As a paint pigment
Metaphosphate	In glasses, porcelain, and enamels
Molybdate	In electronic and optical equipment, as a pigment in paints and protective coatings
Nitrate	In pyrotechnics (green light); in incendiaries; chemicals (barium peroxide); ceramic glazes; as a rodenticide; in vacuum-tube industry
Nitrite	In diazotization reactions; for the prevention of corrosion of steel bars; in explosives
Oxalate	As an analytical reagent; in pyrotechnics
Oxide	As a dehydrating agent; in the manufacture of lubricating oil detergents
Perchlorate	In explosives; in rocket fuels (experimentally); in the determination of ribonuclease; as an absorbent of water in C and H analysis
Permanganate	As a strong disinfectant; in the manufacture of permanganates; as a dry cell depolarizer
Peroxide	In bleach; decolorizing glass; thermal welding of aluminum; in the manufacture of hydrogen peroxide and oxygen in cathodes; in dyeing and printing textiles; as an oxidizing agent in organic synthesis
Phosphate, secondary	In fireproofing compositions; in the preparation of phosphors
Potassium chromate	As a component of anticorrosive paints for use on iron, steel, and light metal alloys
Selenide	In photocells; in semiconductors
Silicate	In refining sugar from molasses
Sodium niobate	In lasers, electro-optical modulators, and optical parametric oscillators
Stearate	As a waterproofing agent; as a lubricant in metalworking, plastics, and rubber; in wax compounding; in the preparation of greases; as a heat and light stabilizer in plastics

Sources in the Environment

Table 4 (contd).

Barium compound	Uses
Sulfate	As weighting mud in oil-drilling; in paper coatings; in paints; as filler and delustrant for textiles, rubber, linoleum, oilcloth, plastics, and lithograph inks; as base for lake colours; as X-ray contrast medium; as opaque medium for gastrointestinal radiography; in battery plate expanders, radiation shields, photographic paper, artificial ivory, cellophane; in heavy concrete for radiation shields
Sulfide	In luminous paint; as a depilatory; as a fireproofing agent; in barium salts; in vulcanizing rubber; in the manufacture of lithopone; in generating pure hydrogen sulfide for analytical purposes; as the main starting material for the production of most barium compounds
Sulfite	In analysis; in the manufacture of paper
Tartrate	In pyrotechnics
Thiocyanate	To make aluminum or potassium thiocyanates; in dyeing; in photography; as a dispersing agent for cellulose
Thiosulfate	In explosives, luminous paints, matches, varnishes; as an iodometry standard; in photographic diffusion-transfer processes.
Titanate (IV)	In ferroelectric ceramic; pure or combined with iron, used in electronic storage devices, dielectric amplifiers, digital calculators, memory devices, and magnetic amplifiers
Tungstate	As a pigment; in X-ray photography for the manufacture of intensifying and phosphorescent screens
Zirconate	In the manufacture of silicone rubber compounds stable up to 246 °C; in electronics
Zirconium silicate	In the production of electrical resistor ceramics and glaze opacifiers; as a stabilizer for coloured ground coat enamels

[a] Source: Hawley (1977), Windholz (1983), Shreve (1967).

Complexes of barium with other compounds are used as additives, which act as dispersants, stabilizers, and inhibitors in several kinds of oils. A barium-based organometallic compound is used to reduce stack smoke emissions from diesel engines. Miner (1969) estimated the amount of barium emitted in diesel exhaust to be a maximum of 12 mg/m^3 ($\leq$25% soluble barium at full load). This estimate was based on the presence of an additive concentration in diesel fuel of 0.075% barium by weight.

Barium compounds are used in the electronics and computer industries, as contrast media in roentgenography, in sugar processing, and as an ingredient in various products such as cosmetics, cloth, leather, linoleum, oil cloth, plastics, pharmaceuticals, printer's ink, photographic paper, depilatories, pyrotechnics, detergents, high-temperature greases, and water softeners (US Bureau of Mines, 1976).

The manufacture of paint also uses barium compounds, including the sulfate, carbonate, and lithopone (a white pigment consisting of a mixture of zinc sulfide, barium sulfate, and zinc oxide). These compounds are relatively unreactive, and their most important pigment properties are high specific gravity, relatively low oil absorption, and easy wettability by oils and grinding agents. The amount of barium that these products add to the environment has not been determined, but most atmospheric emissions are related to material handling (US Bureau of Mines, 1976).

One of the routinely used technologies for treating radium-containing water is to precipitate the radium as barium-radium sulfate or adsorb it on materials containing natural or activated barium sulfate (Havlik et al., 1980).

4. ENVIRONMENTAL TRANSPORT AND DISTRIBUTION

4.1 Transport and distribution between media

4.1.1 Air

Examination of dust falls and suspended particulates indicates that most contain barium. The presence of barium is mainly attributable to industrial emissions, especially the combustion of coal and diesel oil and waste incineration, and may also result from dusts blown from soils and mining processes. Barium sulfate and carbonate are the forms of barium most likely to occur in particulate matter in the air, although the presence of other insoluble compounds cannot be excluded. The residence time of barium in the atmosphere may be several days, depending on the particle size. Most of these particles, however, are much larger than 10 μm in size, and rapidly settle back to earth.

Particles can be removed from the atmosphere by rain-out or wash-out wet deposition. These two forms of deposition efficiently clear the atmosphere of pollutants, but they are not well understood. Without knowing the amount of barium in the atmosphere, it is difficult to evaluate the processes of deposition, transport, and distribution.

4.1.2 Water

Soluble barium and suspended particulates can be transported great distances in rivers, depending on the rates of flow and sedimentation. In the absence of any possible removal mechanisms, the residence time of barium in aquatic systems could be several hundred years. Cartwright et al. (1978) studied the chemical control of barium solubility and showed that for most water samples, barium ion concentration is controlled by the amount of sulfate ion in the water.

Unless it is removed by precipitation, exchange with soil, or other processes, barium in surface waters ultimately reaches the ocean. Once freshwater sources discharge into sea water, barium and the sulfate ions present in salt water form barium sulfate. Due to the relatively higher concentration of sulfate present in the oceans, only an estimated 0.006% of the total barium brought by freshwater sources remains in solution (Chow et al., 1978). This estimate is supported by evidence that outer shelf sediments have lower barium concentrations than those closer to the mainland.

Upon entering the ocean, barium is transported downward by the physical processes of mixing. It is depleted in the upper layers of the ocean by incorporation into biological matter, which settles toward the ocean floor (Goldberg & Arrhenius, 1958). The higher concentration of barium in deep water relative to surface water probably reflects the deposition of barium onto suspended particles forming at the ocean surface and the subsequent release of barium to the deep water as the particles are destroyed in transit to the ocean floor. In the ocean, barium is in steady state; the amount entering the ocean through rivers is balanced by the amount falling to the bottom as particles forming a permanent part of the sediment (Wolgemuth & Brocker, 1970).

4.1.3 Soil

Barium is present in the soil through the natural process of soil formation, which includes the breakdown of parent rocks by weathering. Barium levels are high in soils formed from limestone, feldspar, and biotite micas of the schists and shales (Clark & Washington, 1924). When soluble barium-containing minerals weather and come into contact with solutions containing sulfates, barium sulfate is deposited in available geological faults. If there is insufficient sulfate to combine with barium, the soil material formed is partially saturated with barium. Barium replaces other cations in the soil particles by ion exchange.

Barium salts are preferentially absorbed by argillaceous elements. Colloidal clays have been found to decompose insoluble barium sulfate by binding barium. Bradfield (1932) found that, in the reaction between purified sodium clay and barium sulfate, the sulfate ion became much more soluble, thus releasing the barium into the clay.

Barium in soils would not be expected to be very mobile because of the formation of water-insoluble salts and its inability to form soluble complexes with humic and fulvic materials. Under acid conditions, however, some of the water-insoluble barium compounds may become soluble and move into ground water (US EPA, 1984).

4.1.4 Vegetation and wildlife

Despite relatively high concentrations in soils, only a limited amount of barium accumulates in plants. Barium is actively taken up by legumes, grain stalks, forage plants, red ash leaves, and the black walnut, hickory, and brazil nut trees. The Douglas fir tree and plants of the genus *Astragallu* also accumulate barium. No studies of barium particle uptake from the air have been reported, although vegetation is capable of removing significant amounts of contaminants from the atmosphere. Plant leaves act only as deposition sites for particulate matter. There is no evidence that barium is an essential element in plants (Reeves, 1979).

No information is available on barium levels in wildlife.

4.1.5 Entry into the food chain

Certain plants used by humans as food sources actively accumulate barium. It is also found in dairy products and eggs (Gormican, 1970).

4.2 Biotransformation

There is no evidence that barium undergoes biotransformation other than as a divalent cation.

5. ENVIRONMENTAL LEVELS AND HUMAN EXPOSURE

5.1 Environmental levels

Environmental levels are generally reported as total barium ion rather than as specific barium compounds.

5.1.1 Air

The levels of barium in the air are not well documented, and in some cases the results are contradictory. Tabor & Warren (1958) detected barium concentrations from ≤ 0.005 to 1.5 $\mu g/m^3$ in the air in 18 cities and 4 suburban areas in the USA (Table 5). Of 754 samples analysed, most of the observations made were at concentrations up to 0.05 $\mu g/m^3$. No distinct pattern between ambient levels of barium in the air and the extent of industrialization was observed. In general, however, a higher concentration was observed in areas where metal smelting occurred (Tabor & Warren, 1958; Schroeder, 1970). In a more recent survey in the USA, barium concentration ranged from 0.0015 to 0.95 $\mu g/m^3$ (US EPA, 1984).

In three communities in New York City, barium was measured in dustfall and household dust (Creason et al., 1975). With standard methods (US EPA, 1974), the dustfall was found to contain an average of 137 μg barium/g dust, while the house dust contained 20 μg barium/g.

5.1.2 Water

The presence of barium in sea water, river water, and well water has been well documented. It occurs in almost all surface waters that have been examined (NAS, 1977). The concentration present is extremely variable and depends on factors (e.g., local geology) that affect aquifers and any water treatment that has occurred. The concentration of barium in water is related to the hardness of the water, which is defined as the sum of the polyvalent cations present, including the ions of calcium, magnesium, iron, manganese, copper, barium, and zinc (NAS, 1977). Barium concentrations of 7 to 15 000 μg/litre have

Table 5. Barium in the ambient air of various cities in the USA[a]

City	Percentage of samples at various concentrations (µg/m³)			
	≤ 0.005	> 0.005-0.05	> 0.05-0.5	> 0.5-1.5
Houston (urban, suburban)	24	60	10	6
Boston (urban), Chicago, Denver, E. St. Louis, Louisville, Minneapolis, New Orleans, Portland, Salt Lake City, Tampa	32	52	16	0
Boston (suburban), Chattanooga, E. Chicago, Washington, DC	36	64	0	0
Fort Worth, Jersey City, New York, Philadelphia,	66	34	0	0
Lakehurst (NJ), Paulsboro (NJ) (suburban)	100	0	0	0

[a] Source: Tabor & Warren (1958)

been measured in fresh water and 6 µg/litre in sea water (Schroeder et al., 1972).

5.1.2.1 Surface waters

In the USA, levels of barium in water vary greatly depending on local geochemical influences. Levels reported in various studies are shown in Table 6.

Table 6. Barium content in USA surface waters

Source	Barium Concentration (µg/litre) Range	Mean	Reference
Fresh water	7-15 000	50	Schroeder (1970)
River water	9-150	57 (54 median)	Durum (1960)
Surface water	2-340	43	Kopp (1969); Kopp & Kroner (1970)
Surface water	10-12 000	50	Bradford (1971)

5.1.2.2 Drinking-water

Municipal water supplies depend upon the quality of surface waters and ground waters, and these, in turn, depend upon local geochemical influences. Studies of the water quality in cities in the USA have revealed levels of barium ranging from a trace to 10 000 µg/litre (Durfor & Becker, 1964; Barnett et al., 1969; McCabe et al., 1970; McCabe, 1974; Calabrese, 1977; AWWA, 1985). Drinking-water levels of at least 1000 µg barium/litre have been reported when the barium is present mainly in the form of insoluble salts (Kojola et al., 1978). Levels of barium in Canadian water supplies have been reported to range from 5 to 600 µg/litre (Subramanian & Meranger, 1984), and municipal water levels in Sweden ranging from 1 to 20 µg/litre have been measured (Reeves, 1986).

5.1.2.3 Ocean waters

The concentration of barium in sea water varies greatly with factors such as latitude, depth, and the ocean in question. Several studies have shown that the barium content in the open ocean increases with the depth of water (Chow & Goldberg, 1960; Bolter et al., 1964; Turekian, 1965; Chow & Patterson, 1966; Anderson & Hume, 1968). A Geosecs III study of the southwest Pacific by Bacon & Edmond (1972) found a barium profile of 4.9 µg/litre in surface waters to 19.5 µg/litre in deep waters. Later studies by Chow (1976) and Chow et al. (1978) corroborated these values. The barium concentration in the northeast Pacific ranges from 8.5 to 32 µg/litre (Wolgemuth & Brocker, 1970). Bernat et al. (1972) found that barium concentration profiles for the eastern Pacific Ocean and the Mediterranean Sea ranged from 5.2 to 25.2 µg/litre and from 10.6 to 12.7 µg/litre, respectively.

Anderson & Hume (1968) reported concentrations in the Atlantic Ocean ranging from 0.8 to 37.0 µg/litre in the equatorial region and from 0.04 to 22.8 µg/litre in the North Atlantic, with mean values of 6.5 and 7.6 µg/litre, respectively. In Atlantic Ocean waters off Bermuda, barium concentrations of 15.9-19.1 µg/litre have been measured (Chow & Patterson, 1966).

5.1.3 Soil and sediment

The presence of barium in soils has received attention since it was first documented in the muds of the River Nile (Knop, 1874) and the soils of the USA (Crawford, 1908). In the earth's crust the barium concentration is 400 to 500 mg/kg (Wells, 1937; Schroeder, 1970; Davis, 1972). Later works have verified the levels found in the early studies. The background level of barium in soils is considered to range from 100 to 3000 mg/kg, the average abundance being 500 mg/kg (Brooks, 1978).

The concentrations of barium in sediments of the Iowa river are 450 to 3000 mg/kg (Tsai et al., 1978), suggesting that barium in the water is removed by precipitation and silting and may possibly affect the ecology of benthic organisms.

5.1.4 Food

A review of the early literature summarizes the quantity of barium present in many plants (Robinson et al.,

1950). Barium has been found in grain stalks, forage plants, red ash leaves, and in the black walnut, hickory, and Brazil nut trees. With the exception of the Brazil nut tree, those parts of the plants that accumulate barium are seldom eaten by man. Various studies document the concentrations of barium in Brazil nuts ranging from 1500-3000 mg/kg (Robinson et al., 1950; Smith, 1971a). Barium is also present in wheat, although most is concentrated in the stalks and leaves rather than in the grain (Smith, 1971b). Tomatoes and soybeans also concentrate soil barium, the bioconcentration factor ranging from 2 to 20 (Robinson et al., 1950). Gormican (1970) determined the barium content of a large number of food items, including dairy products, cereals, fruits and vegetables, and meats (Table 7). In the beverages group, tea and cocoa had the highest barium content (2.7 and 1.2 mg/100 g, respectively) on a dry-weight basis. Among breads, cereal products, and cracker products, bran flakes (0.39 mg/100 g) and enriched instant cream of wheat (0.2 mg/100 g) had the highest levels. Eggs were found to have 0.76 mg/100 g, and swiss cheese 0.22 mg/100 g. Fruits and fruit juice had low barium levels, the highest values being in raw, unpeeled apples (0.075 mg/100 g). These levels are similar to those found in grapes (<0.05 mg/100 g) and cooked prunes (0.064 mg/100 g). All meats showed concentrations of 0.04 mg per 100 g or less. Vegetables had relatively low barium levels, with the exception of beets (0.26 mg/100 g) and sweet potatoes (0.22 mg/100 g). Among nuts, pecans had the highest barium content (0.67 mg/100 g).

5.1.5 Feed

Barium generally does not accumulate in common plants in sufficient quantities to be toxic to animals. However, Robinson et al. (1950) suggested that the large quantities of barium (as high as 1260 mg/kg) accumulating in legumes, alfalfa, and soybeans grown in soils containing high exchangeable barium content may cause problems in domestic cattle.

5.1.6 Other products

McHargue (1913) reported that the barium content of dry tobacco leaves was in the range 88-293 mg/kg. Later

Table 7. Barium contents of some common foods[a]

Food	Barium content (mg/100 g)
Beverages and dietary concentrates	
Chocolate syrup	0.17
Coffee	
Instant, dry	0.36
Ground, dry	0.32
Beverage, brewed	<0.008
Cocoa, dry	1.2
Meritene, plain flavour, dry	0.11
Sustagen, imitation vanilla flavour	0.056
Tea, orange pekoe	
Bag, dry	2.7
Beverage, steeped	<0.004
Breads, cereal products, crackers, and pastas	
Bread	
Rye	0.062
White	0.051
Whole wheat	0.11
Bran flakes, 40%	0.39
Cheerios (cereal)	0.13
Corn flakes (cereal)	0.04
Crackers	
Graham	0.11
Saltines	0.04
Egg noodles, uncooked	0.16
Macaroni, uncooked	0.11
Oatmeal, rolled oats (quick), uncooked	0.11
Puffed Rice	<0.04
Quick Cream of Wheat (cereal)	
Enriched, uncooked	0.2
Regular, uncooked	0.15
Rice Krispies	<0.04
Rice, white uncooked	<0.04
Shredded Wheat	0.22
Wheaties (cereal)	0.14
Spaghetti, uncooked	0.11
Cheese	
American	0.12
Cottage, creamed	<0.04
Swiss	0.22
Eggs	
Whole	0.76
White	<0.01
Yolk	0.058
Milk	
Nonfat solids	<0.08

Table 7 (contd).

Food	Barium content (mg/100 g)
Milk (contd).	
Fluid	
Whole	<0.01
Skim	<0.01
Buttermilk	<0.01
Ice cream, vanilla	<0.01
Sherbet, orange	<0.01
Fruits and fruit juices	
Apple	
Raw, unpeeled	0.075
Juice, canned	<0.002
Sauce, canned, drained	<0.01
Apricots, canned, drained	<0.01
Banana, ripe	<0.01
Blueberries, waterpack, drained	0.014
Cantaloupe	<0.01
Cherries, Royal Anne, canned, drained	0.029
Grapes	
Fresh, with peel	<0.05
Juice, canned	0.023
Grapefruit	
Juice, canned	<0.008
Sections	
Fresh, skinless	<0.01
Canned, drained	<0.01
Orange	
Juice, frozen, reconstituted	<0.008
Sections, skinless	<0.008
Pineapple	
Crushed, canned, drained	0.014
Juice, canned	0.008
Peach, cling, canned, drained	<0.01
Pear, canned, drained	0.047
Prunes	
Cooked	0.064
Juice	0.014
Watermelon	0.022
Meat, poultry, fish, and shellfish	
Beef, fresh, uncooked	
Flank, round, rump, sirloin, or tenderloin	<0.02
Ground	<0.02
Liver	<0.04
Lamb, fresh, uncooked	
Chop	<0.02
Leg	<0.02
Luncheon meat, big bologna	<0.02
Pork, fresh, uncooked	

Table 7 (contd).

Food	Barium content (mg/100 g)
Meat, poultry, fish, and shellfish (contd).	
Bacon	<0.04
Ham	<0.02
Liver	<0.04
Loin	<0.02
Veal, fresh, uncooked	
Round or steak	<0.02
Poultry, uncooked	
Chicken, roaster	
Dark meat	<0.02
White meat	<0.02
Turkey, roaster	
Dark meat	<0.02
White meat	<0.02
Fish and shellfish	
Crab, haddock, salmon, sockeye, sole, or tuna	<0.02
Shrimp	<0.02
Nuts	
Peanuts	
Butter	<0.04
Salted, blanched	0.21
Pecans	0.67
Walnuts	0.072
Sugars and flours	
Sugar	
Brown	<0.04
Powdered	<0.04
White	<0.04
Flour, bleached, enriched	0.072
Vegetables	
Asparagus spears, frozen, uncooked	<0.02
Beans	
Baked with pork	<0.02
Green, frozen, uncooked	0.16
Lima, baby, frozen, uncooked	0.031
Wax, canned, salt-free, drained	0.11
Beets, canned, salt-free, drained	0.26
Broccoli, frozen, uncooked	<0.02
Brussels sprouts, frozen, uncooked	<0.02
Cabbage, uncooked	<0.02
Carrots, uncooked	0.052
Cauliflower, frozen, uncooked	<0.02
Celery, fresh	<0.02
Corn, whole kernel, canned, salt-free, drained	<0.02
Cucumber	<0.02

Table 7 (contd).

Food	Barium content (mg/100 g)
Vegetables (contd).	
Lettuce	<0.02
Mushrooms, stems and pieces, canned	<0.02
Onions, fresh, mature	0.053
Peas, canned, salt-free, drained	<0.02
Potato	
Fresh, uncooked	<0.02
Instant, uncooked	0.056
Pumpkin, canned	0.053
Spinach, frozen, uncooked	0.04
Squash, frozen, cooked	0.083
Sweet potatoes, canned	0.22
Tomato	
Fresh	<0.02
Juice, canned, salt-free	<0.008

[a] Source: Gormican (1970)

measurements yielded 24-170 mg/kg, with an average value of 105 mg/kg (Voss & Nicol, 1960). Most of this barium is likely to remain in the ash during burning. The concentrations of barium in tobacco smoke have not been reported.

Bowen (1956) reported the following levels of barium in plants: 15 mg/kg dry weight in plankton; 31 mg/kg dry weight in brown algae; 18 mg/kg dry weight in ferns; and 14 mg/kg dry weight in angiosperms.

5.1.7 Nuclear fallout

The principal potential source of radioactive isotopes of barium is nuclear weapons testing. Atmospheric testing suspends radioactive dusts in the upper troposphere where, depending on atmospheric conditions, dusts are carried around the world several times.

The lightest dust particles reach the stratosphere. Several years are required for the bulk of this radioactive material to be deposited on the ground. Since 1952, when tests began on nuclear weapons with high explosive yields, fall-out from the stratosphere has been more or less continuous. Most of this nuclear fall-out occurs in the temperate and polar regions of the earth. The total radiation from nuclear testing has added 10-15% to the naturally occurring radiation throughout the world.

Because ^{140}Ba and ^{143}Ba are radioactive by-products of the thermal nuclear fission of ^{235}U, their concentration in the environment increases after the detonation of a nuclear device in the atmosphere. After a single atmospheric nuclear detonation in China, Gudiksen et al. (1965) detected ^{140}Ba at an altitude of 10 670 m at levels of 177-530 x 10^6 atoms/m^3 over north-western USA. This far exceeds the levels normally present in the atmosphere.

Radioactive particles are normally cleared from the atmosphere by rain and snow. Cooper et al. (1970) monitored ^{140}Ba concentrations in rain and snow in 772 samples collected between 1958 and 1969 and found that debris containing ^{140}Ba was deposited after the atmospheric testing of nuclear weapons in China. Evans et al. (1973) reported the atmospheric level of barium, 4 days after a test in China, to be 4.5 pCi/m^3, which is approximately 30 times higher than the normal background level (0.14 pCi/m^3).

5.2 General population exposure

5.2.1 Environmental sources, food, drinking-water, and air

The most important route of exposure to barium appears to be ingestion of barium through drinking-water and food. Particles containing barium may be inhaled into the lung, but little is known regarding the absorption of barium by this route.

In studies of dietary intake in two hospitals, 300 schools, and individual subjects in the USA, Underwood (1977) determined that the average intake of barium ranged from 300 to 1700 µg/day. An earlier study had found that the barium intake from diets served to adults in American hospitals in the summer was not more than 303 µg/day and in winter not more than 592 µg/day (Gormican, 1970).

Tipton et al. (1966, 1969) studied five adult subjects whose self-selected diets were examined for varying lengths of time. Barium concentrations were measured in all foods consumed for 30 days by two subjects, 70 days by one other, and 347 days by the remaining two subjects. Intakes of barium showed large variations and ranged from 650 to 1770 µg/day.

In the United Kingdom, the total intake of barium from the diet was estimated by Hamilton & Minski (1972) to be approximately 603 µg/day and by the ICRP (1959) to be 900 µg/day. Schroeder et al. (1972) estimated that the mean daily intake of barium in food is 1.24 mg, in water 0.086 mg, and in air 0.001 mg, giving a total of 1.33 mg/day. The ICRP (1974) reported the dietary intake of barium to be 0.75 mg/day, including both food and fluids. The contribution from drinking-water was estimated to be about 0.08 mg/day, which leaves 0.67 mg/day from other dietary sources. When Murphy et al. (1971) analysed school lunches from 300 schools in 19 states in the USA, the barium content ranged from 0.09 to 0.43 mg/lunch, with a mean of 0.17 mg. Milk, potatoes, and flour have been suggested to be the major sources of barium in diets in the USA (Calabrese et al., 1985).

The barium content in drinking-water seems to depend on regional geochemical conditions. In a study of the water supplies of the 100 largest cities in the USA, a median value of 43 µg/litre was reported; 94% of all determinations were $\leq$100 µg/litre (Durfor & Becker, 1964). This represents an average intake of $\leq$200 µg/day.

More recent studies by Letkiewicz et al. (1984) indicated that approximately 214 million people in the USA using public water supplies are exposed to barium levels ranging from 1 to 20 µg/litre. In certain regions of the USA, however, barium may reach 10 000 µg/litre. In these areas, the average intake could be as high as 20 000 µg/day (Calabrese, 1977).

Drinking-water appears to be an important source of human exposure to barium. The digestive system is extremely permeable to soluble barium, allowing rapid absorption into (and removal from) the bloodstream (Castagnou et al., 1957). This is important when considering uptake of barium from drinking-water, since a large percentage of barium in water is in the soluble form.

Due to the paucity of information on the ambient levels of barium in the air, it is difficult to estimate the intake from this source. As described earlier (section 5.1.3), the levels of barium in air rarely exceed 0.05 µg/m³ (Tabor & Warren, 1958). This value can be used to estimate daily barium intake via the lungs. Assuming that the average lung ventilation (LV) rate for newborn babies, male adults undergoing light activity, and male adults undergoing heavy activity is 0.5, 20, and 43 litres/min, respectively (ICRP, 1975), the intake via inhalation would range from 0.04 to 3.1 µg/day. Other age groups and females are included in this range. Earlier, the ICRP (1974) reported that intake of barium through inhalation ranges from 0.09 to 26 µg/day.

Because the chemical properties of the barium entering the lung are not known, it is difficult to ascertain the amount retained. Retention in adult animals is approximately 20% (Cuddihy & Ozog, 1973), which suggests that insoluble barium accumulates and is slowly removed.

Another source of exposure is radioactive isotopes of barium from nuclear fall-out after the explosion of nuclear weapons. ^{140}Ba and ^{143}Ba are the main radioactive products of the thermal-nuclear fission of ^{235}U, and their half-lives are 12.8 days and 12 seconds, respectively (CRC, 1988). Therefore, the potential for exposure depends on its presence at ground level (air, soil, water contamination), as well as on the time elapsed since explosion. In terms of biochemical and pharmacological effects, the exposure to barium from this source is not significant. However, because exposure to radioactive isotopes results in bone deposition, retention may be a concern.

5.2.2 Other sources

Barium sulfate is the major barium compound used medicinally. This very poorly soluble compound is employed as an opaque contrast medium for roentgenographic studies of the gastrointestinal tract. There is limited evidence that the ingestion of the compound may cause deleterious biological effects. However, one study suggested that radiation-induced gastrointestinal effects may be reduced by the ingestion of barium sulfate (Conard & Scott, 1961).

5.2.3 Subpopulations at special risk

Patients receiving drugs such as acetazolamide (glaucoma treatment; diuretic agent) or thiazide diuretics have increased urinary potassium excretion ($\leq$60% and 400%, respectively) and would be at higher risk of potassium deficiency due to barium toxicity. Patients subject to X-ray studies of the gastrointestinal tract have shown occasional increases in serum protein-bound iodine (PBI) (Wallach, 1978).

5.3 Occupational exposure during manufacture, formulation, or use

The US National Institute for Occupational Safety and Health (NIOSH) has investigated occupational exposures to barium in a variety of industrial operations in response to requests submitted by employers and workers for health hazard evaluations and technical assistance. Table 8 summarizes the exposures and adverse health effects found in these investigations.

Occupational exposure to soluble barium compounds has been reported for workers exposed to welding fumes (Dare et al., 1984). The wiring used in arc welding processes was shown to contain 20-40% soluble barium compounds, and fumes produced during these processes contained 25% barium. Urine analysis of workers revealed barium concentrations ranging from 31 to 234 µg/litre after 3 h of exposure. Follow-up samples taken approximately 12 h after exposure contained levels ranging from 20 to 110 µg/litre. The level in the urine of controls ranged from 1.8 to 4.7 µg/litre. No air samples were collected, but NIOSH (1978) reported that welders using the same wire were exposed to 2200 to 6200 µg soluble barium per m^3.

Table 8. Occupational exposure to barium in various industries

Industry	Compound	Concentration range, mg/m^3	Number of samples[a]	Health effects	Comments	Reference
Magnetic plastic	BaFe$_{12}$O$_{19}$ Ba (soluble)	< 0.08-2.2 < 0.01-0.27	22	none reported		NIOSH (1976)
Steel, arc welding	Ba (soluble)	2.2-6.1	5	none reported	see Dare et al. (1984)	NIOSH (1978)
Vinyl floor	Ba (soluble)	≤ 0.4	9	none reported		NIOSH (1979)
Metal alloys	Ba (soluble)	0.02-1.7	12	musculoskeletal, gastro-intestinal, skin, respiratory	exposures to lead, zirconim, UV, visible, and IR radiation	NIOSH (1980)
Mineral ores	Ba (soluble)	0.01-1.92	27	hypertension	exposure to lead, zinc	NIOSH (1982)
Petroleum refinery, TCCU turn-around	Ba (soluble)	0.03-0.05 (mean) 0.015-2.50 (max)	NR	none		NIOSH (1984)
Auto parts	Ba (soluble)	0.002-0.68	68	none reported		NIOSH (1985)
Aluminium foundry	Ba (soluble)	0.001-0.037	13	eye, nasal irritation	exposures to silica, formaldehyde	NIOSH (1987a,b,c)
Fire extinguisher	BaO	0.08-1.7	4	none reported	ZnO fumes	NIOSH (1987a,b,c)

[a] NR = not reported.

6. KINETICS AND METABOLISM

6.1 Absorption

Barium enters the body primarily through the inhalation and ingestion processes. The degree of absorption of barium from the lungs and gastrointestinal tract varies according to the animal species, the solubility of the compound, gastrointestinal tract content, and age. Studies with soluble barium salts have shown that these compounds are readily absorbed (Cuddihy & Griffith, 1972; Cuddihy & Ozog, 1973; Cuddihy et al., 1974; McCauley & Washington, 1983). Recent studies have indicated that poorly soluble barium compounds may also be absorbed (McCauley & Washington, 1983; Clavel et al., 1987).

6.1.1 Inhalation route

6.1.1.1 Laboratory animals

Cuddihy & Ozog (1973) studied the absorption of labelled barium chloride ($^{133}BaCl_2$) solutions in 1-year-old Syrian hamsters. Absorption into the general circulation of solutions deposited on nasal membranes was compared with gastrointestinal tract absorption. During the first 4 h after administration, barium absorption from the nasal passages was approximately 61%, compared with 11% gastric absorption. The authors concluded that the nasopharynx is a major absorption site for inhaled aerosols of soluble barium, especially for readily soluble aerosols having mass median aerodynamic diameters >5 μm.

Gutwein et al. (1974) observed that on day 24 after the exposure of male Sprague-Dawley rats (275 g) by nasal intubation to combustion products from diesel fuel containing a barium-based additive in solution (vehicle not specified), more than 85% of the administered dose was found in the bone, indicating significant absorption in the respiratory tract.

The principle mechanism for removing insoluble particles from the lung is transport by the ciliated epithelium and its associated mucosal lining, followed by swallowing. Spritzer & Watson (1964) evaluated the ciliary clearance of poorly soluble barium sulfate and found that 52% of the compound introduced into rat lung was removed by ciliary action. The other 48% was removed by "lung-to-blood transfer mechanisms" (probably macrophage activity), which led to disposal of the sulfate particles. These mechanisms suggest that solubilization of the barium sulfate occurs *in vivo*.

Clearance from the lungs of various forms of barium after inhalation exposure of rats and beagle dogs was studied by Einbrodt et al. (1972) and Cuddihy et al. (1974). Einbrodt et al. (1972) exposed rats to barium sulfate (40 mg/m^3) for 2 months, and this was followed by a 4-week observation interval. Animals were killed at 2-week intervals. After 2 weeks of exposure, the barium content in the lungs was high but decreased rapidly over the next 4 weeks of exposure and then increased again during the observation period. Barium accumulation in bone tissue increased initially, but with continued exposure decreased. There was no absorption into lymph tissue.

In beagle dogs exposed to various barium compounds (chloride, sulfate, heat-treated sulfate, or barium in fused montmorillonite clay), barium was cleared from the lungs at a rate of proportional to its solubility (Cuddihy et al., 1974). The longest retention time in the lungs was for barium adsorbed to clay; more than 500 days after exposure, 10% of the initial body burden was still in the lungs and skeleton (Cuddihy et al., 1974). For barium sulfate, there was a long-term slow clearance, with virtually no change in lung tissue levels of barium from 8 to 16 days after exposure. The clearance rate depended on the specific surface area of the inhaled particles. In Syrian hamsters, barium sulfate was found to be cleared from the lungs with a biological half-life of 8-9 days (Morrow et al., 1964). This indicated some dispersion of barium sulfate in body fluids, possibly in a colloidal form.

6.1.1.2 *Humans*

There are no quantitative data on the deposition and absorption of barium compounds through inhalation in humans.

6.1.2 Oral route

6.1.2.1 Laboratory animals

The absorption of ingested barium depends on factors such as the presence of food in the intestine, the sulfate content in the food, the age of the animal, and the location of the barium in the gastrointestinal tract. Absorption of barium from the gastrointestinal tract has been studied in rats (Taylor et al., 1962). Labelled barium chloride was administered by intragastric intubation to groups of 5-10 brown-hooded female rats (14 days to 70 weeks old). Absorption was estimated as the radioactivity 7 h after exposure in the carcass plus urine minus gastrointestinal tract in relation to the dose. The absorption decreased with age, from approximately 85% of the administered dose at 14-18 days of age, to 63% at 22 days, to approximately 7% after 6-8 or 60-70 weeks of age. Deprivation of food before administration (18 h) markedly increased the absorption of barium, from approximately 7% in fed animals to 20% in fasted animals 6-8 or 60-70 weeks old. Administration of the compound in cow's milk did not affect absorption.

In studies by Cuddihy & Ozog (1973), groups of 5-10 Syrian hamsters (1 year old) were administered labelled barium chloride by intragastric intubation. The absorption estimate was based on carcass radioactivity 4 h after exposure in relation to carcass radioactivity immediately after intravenous administration (100%). Results show that following a 12 h fasting, a combination of gastric (32%) and intestinal (11%) absorption was found during the first 4 h after administration. McCauley & Washington (1983) examined the absorption of specific barium salt anions in male Sprague-Dawley rats, administering radiolabelled barium chloride, sulfate, or carbonate to fasted (24 h) and non-fasted rats by gastric intubation. Animals were sacrificed from 2 to 480 min after administration and blood concentrations were measured. In general, barium blood concentrations were higher in fasted animals and reached a peak 15 min after dosing, whereas non-fasted animals had lower barium blood concentrations and peaked 60 min after dosing. The peak blood concentrations of the carbonate and sulfate salts were 45% and 85%, respectively, of that of the chloride.

Orally administered barium chloride ($^{133}BaCl_2$) was found to be rapidly absorbed from the gastrointestinal tract of male weanling rats, the peak concentration in the bloodstream and soft tissues occurring 30 min after dosing. Total uptake of barium increased with increasing dosage, but, there appeared to be a saturation point for oral absorption (Clary & Tardiff, 1974).

6.1.2.2 Humans

There are few data on the absorption of barium from the human gastrointestinal tract. Tipton et al. (1969) reported that two males fed controlled diets for 80 weeks absorbed between 2 and 6% of the barium content in their diet, based on urinary elimination. Elimination via the gastrointestinal tract was not given. Recent studies by Clavel et al. (1987) have shown that insoluble barium salts commonly used during radiological investigations are absorbed by the intestine and are excreted in the urine.

6.1.3 Parenteral administration

The *in vivo* solubility of four barium compounds (the chloride, sulfate, and carbonate salts and fused clay forms of previously aerosolized material resuspended in distilled water) was studied in rats after intramuscular injection (Thomas et al., 1973). The chloride and carbonate salts were found to be equally soluble in the soft tissues and were absorbed from the injection site very rapidly.

6.2 Distribution

6.2.1 Levels in tissues of experimental animals

Studies in rats and mice have shown that barium is incorporated into the bone matrix in much the same way as calcium (Bauer et al., 1956; Taylor et al., 1962; Bligh & Taylor, 1963; Domanski et al., 1969; Dencker et al., 1976). This means that the major part of the body burden will be in the skeleton. Soft tissues generally have low concentrations of barium, an exception being pig-mented areas of the eye (Sowden & Pirie, 1958). Barium is incorporated into the bone, especially in young animals that are still growing. In mature animals, 60-80% of the barium initially deposited is removed from the femur during the first 14 days after exposure (Bligh & Taylor, 1963). The uptake of barium into bone decreases with the age of the animal. No detrimental effects on the integrity of the bone have been seen.

Dencker et al. (1976) injected labelled barium chloride ($^{133}BaCl_2$) intravenously in pigmented and albino mice (63 µg barium/kg body weight). Autoradiography revealed that uptake was rapid and retention times were longest in calcified tissues, cartilage, and melanin-containing tissues. In other tissues, the radioactivity rapidly disappeared. In the mouse fetus, the authors found that barium is mainly taken up by the skeleton, especially in the growth zones. Except for the eye, soft tissues had a low uptake.

Barium deposition appears to occur preferentially in the most active areas of bone growth (Bligh & Taylor, 1963), although research indicates that the preferential uptake of barium is localized primarily in the periosteal, endosteal, and trabular surfaces of the bone (Ellsasser et al., 1969).

McCauley & Washington (1983) found that 24 h after an intragastric dose of labelled barium chloride to rats, the highest concentration was in the heart, followed by the eye, kidney, liver, and blood. Clary & Tardiff (1974) found that labelled barium chloride ($^{133}BaCl_2$) administered orally to weanling male rats entered the bloodstream and soft tissues, peak concentrations occurring 30 min after administration. Uptake was observed in the submaxillary salivary gland, adrenal gland, kidney, gastric mucosa, and blood vessels. The deposition of barium in hard tissues was detected after 2 h. In a more recent study, Tardiff et al. (1980) administered barium chloride (10, 50, or 250 mg barium/litre of drinking-water) to young adult rats of both sexes for 4, 8, or 13 weeks. Barium deposition in liver, skeletal muscle, heart, and bone was dose-dependent but not related to the length of exposure. The highest concentration of barium was observed in the bones. In the soft tissues, concentrations were <1 mg/kg even after 13 weeks of exposure to 250 mg barium per litre. In the bone, the average concentration was 226 mg/kg.

In dogs, inhalation of radioactive barium (the chloride or sulfate salts) resulted in significant (when compared to other tissues) radioactive deposition in the bone (chloride) and in the lung (sulfate) (Cuddihy & Griffith, 1972). Rats that inhaled 40 mg barium sulfate over a 2-month period initially accumulated barium in their bones (jaw and femur). However, the rate of deposition decreased with continued exposure (Einbrodt et al., 1972). Similarly, 2 weeks after the initiation of exposure, lung barium content was high, whereas it decreased over the next 4 weeks but increased again during 4 weeks in the post-inhalation period. No evidence for the transport of barium in lymph was noted by these authors.

6.2.2 Levels in human tissue

It has been estimated that the "Standard Man" (a term borrowed from radiation dosimetry) of 70 kg contains approximately 22 mg of barium (Tipton et al., 1963). A major part of the element is concentrated in the bone (nearly 91%), the remainder being in soft tissues such as the aorta, brain, heart, kidney, spleen, pancreas, and lung (Schroeder, 1970). In human beings there is no increase of total barium with age, except in the aorta and lung (Venugopal & Luckey, 1978). Sowden & Stitch (1957) reported that uptake of barium into bone did not increase with age (Table 9). Bligh & Taylor (1963) and Ellsasser et al. (1969) found that barium deposition in the bone occurred preferentially in the active sites of bone growth.

Table 9. Concentration of barium in human bone ($\mu g/g$) according to age[a]

	0-3 months	1-13 years	19-33 years	33-74 years
No. of subjects	7	9	9	10
Concentration range	1.9-13.0	2.1-21.0	4.3-7.9	3.7-17.3
Mean	7.0	7.7	5.1	8.5
Standard deviation	± 4.0	± 7.0	± 0.12	± 4.0

[a] Source: Bligh & Taylor (1963).

In the USA, the highest concentration in soft tissues was found in the large intestine, muscle, and lung. The median values were approximately 0.15 mg/kg wet weight (Tipton & Cook, 1963; Tipton et al., 1965; Schroeder et al., 1972). In the liver and kidney, the median concentrations were <0.003 and approximately 0.1 mg/kg wet weight, respectively. However, tissue values from subjects from other countries show large differences. The concentration of barium in various tissues was measured in autopsied subjects from the USA, Africa, the Eastern Mediterranean, and South-East Asia (Tipton et al., 1965). For almost all organs examined (aorta, brain, heart, kidney, liver, and spleen), subjects from Africa, the Eastern Mediterranean, and South-East Asia were found to contain higher levels of barium than their counterparts from the USA. In comparison with the other groups, the Eastern Mediterranean group showed higher levels in the lung, and both the Eastern Mediterranean and South-East Asia groups had higher levels in pancreas and testis. Median barium concentrations in liver from people in Africa, the Eastern Mediterranean, South-East Asia, and Switzerland were 0.05, 0.08, 0.05, and 0.02 mg/kg, respectively. The data on subjects in the USA indicated increases with age in certain tissues (e.g., the lung and aorta), whereas the data on subjects from other countries indicated the opposite, except in the case of the lung (Perry et al., 1962).

Harrison et al. (1966) found that whole body retention of barium in humans, 15 days after a single-dose injection of labelled barium chloride ($^{133}BaCl_2$), was 10.5% of the initial dose.

In the USA, barium in the tooth enamel of people under 20 years of age has been found to average 4.2 mg/kg dry weight (Losee et al., 1974), and Cutress (1979) reported a mean barium concentration of 22 mg/kg (a range of 0.8-432 mg/kg) in the teeth of people less than 20 years old from 13 countries. Miller et al. (1985) reported that the mean barium/calcium ratio in teeth was five times higher in 34 children from one community exposed to drinking-water containing an average concentration of 10 mg/litre than that in 35 children from a similar community with much lower levels of barium in the drinking-water (0.2 mg/litre).

Normal levels of barium in hair are generally 1-2 mg/kg (Creason et al., 1975, 1976).

According to Schroeder & Mitchener (1975b), barium has been identified in all samples taken from stillborn babies and children up to one year of age, implying that barium can cross the placental barrier and be transported in the maternal milk.

6.3 Elimination and excretion

The elimination of either injected or ingested barium in both humans and animals occurs principally in the faeces rather than in the urine (Harrison et al., 1967; Domanski et al., 1969; Tipton et al., 1969; Gutwein et al., 1974; Clary & Tardiff, 1974).

6.3.1 Laboratory animals

In young rats given an intraperitoneal dose of carrier-free ^{140}Ba, 18.4% (average of four rats) of the dose had been recovered in the gastrointestinal tract and faeces 4 h after dosing and 5.8% in urine. After 24 h, the corresponding values in three rats were 22.7 and 6.6%. Thus, there was a change from an initial rapid clearance to a slower phase (Bauer et al., 1956). The biological half-time for barium in the bone of mice seems to be 100 days (Dencker et al., 1976), while Clary & Tardiff (1974) estimated the value in the bone of rats to be 90-120 days. According to Domanski et al. (1964), 34.8% of the initial dose was found in rats 16 days after a single-dose injection of barium chloride. In lactating cows, excretion in milk during the first 8 days after dosing was 0.6% of an oral dose and 10% of an intravenously administered dose (Garner et al., 1960). Thomas et al. (1973) reported that in rats barium sulfate disappeared from the injection site with a half-life of 26 days; beyond 100 days the disappearance of barium from bone was similar for both soluble and poorly soluble compounds, the half-life being 460 days.

Gutwein et al. (1974) exposed 14 rats for 10 h to combustion products from fuel to which a barium-containing smoke-suppressant additive (approximately 20% ^{133}BaSO$_4$) was added. Six animals were then killed after radioactive counting. The remaining eight were killed 3-24 days after exposure. Most barium was eliminated via the faeces. The elimination from the lungs was rapid with >50% of the initial lung burden being eliminated during the first 3 days.

6.3.2 Humans

The elimination of barium occurs in both the faeces and the urine, and varies with the route of administration and the solubility of the compound. Within 24 h, 20% of an ingested dose (solubility not specified) appeared in the faeces and 5-7% was excreted in the urine (Venugopal & Luckey, 1978). Furthermore, barium that had been absorbed and transported by the plasma was found to have been almost entirely cleared from the bloodstream within 24 h (Browning, 1969).

In healthy human beings in a state of barium equilibrium (virtually all of the intake occurring by mouth), approximately 91% of the total output was found in the faeces, 6% in sweat, and 3% in urine (Schroeder et al., 1972).

In a study by Harrison et al. (1966), the excretion via the faeces and the urine was measured for 10 days in a healthy 60-year-old man given an intravenous injection of ^{133}Ba. The barium elimination 3-6 h after administration was measured in saliva and seminal fluid, yielding values of 0.22-0.33 and 0.81% of the dose, respectively. The percentage of the injected dose eliminated via the faeces and the urine was 20% after 24 h, 70% after 3 days, and 85% after 10 days. The ratio of faecal to urinary barium was 9.0 after 8 days.

6.4 Metabolism

The mechanisms by which barium is deposited in body tissues are not well characterized. However, the general patterns of uptake show similarities to those of calcium and strontium.

6.4.1 Laboratory animals

In a metabolic study, Bauer et al. (1956) administered intraperitoneal injections of ^{140}Ba and ^{45}Ca to young rats. The results indicated that there was no difference in the metabolism of the two cations. Barium was transferred more rapidly than calcium from the exchangeable to the non-exchangeable fractions of bone, but these differences were not significant. In addition Bligh & Taylor (1963) noted age-related changes in metabolism (Table 9).

7. EFFECTS ON ORGANISMS IN THE ENVIRONMENT

7.1 Microorganisms

7.1.1 Viruses

Various studies have shown that barium can directly influence the physico-chemical properties of viruses as well as their infectivity. At low temperature (5 °C) and concentration (10 mmol/litre), the Ba^{2+} ion, like Mg^{2+} or K^+, causes depolymerization of tobacco mosaic virus protein (McMichael & Lauffer, 1975). Barium and other divalent cations prevent antibiotics such as streptomycin and kanamycin from inhibiting the multiplication of tobacco mosaic virus in protoplasts (Kassanis et al., 1975).

Barium is an effective divalent cation in promoting phage R17 infection (Paranchych, 1966). Divalent cations are essential for the penetration of the phage RNA into the host cell. Ba^{2+} (at concentrations of 0.5-20 mmol per litre) and other divalent cations, e.g., Ca^{2+}, Sr^{2+}, and Mn^{2+}, prevented the haemolysis caused by the infection of chicken erythrocytes with Sendai virus (Toister & Loyter, 1970). These cations may affect virus structure. The calcium ion was reported to be essential for cell fusion by the haemagglutinating virus of Japan (HVJ). When Ca^{2+} was absent, the cells were lysed, not fused, by the virus (Koshi, 1966). Ba^{2+} in equimolar concentration was found to replace Ca^{2+} for this activity.

7.1.2 Bacteria

A number of inorganic elements have been found to be constituents of microorganisms. Not only are these elements firmly bound in various ionic forms and involved in metabolic processes, but they also have a stabilizing effect on the structural integrity of cellular membranes. Spectrochemical analyses of bacterial ash have shown the presence of barium in the following species: *Salmonella paratyphi*, *Salmonella typhosa*, *Shigella flexnerii*, *Shigella dysenteriae*, *Mycobacterium tuberculosis*, and

Vibrio cholerae (Kovalskii et al., 1965). The content of barium was found to be higher in most of the following bacteria than in higher plants: *Escherischia coli, Bacillus cereus, Sphaerotilus natams*, and *Micrococcus roseus* (Rouf, 1964).

Barium, like other divalent cations, maintains the organization and structure of the bacterial cell wall. Addition of Ba^{2+} to osmotically fragile cells of *Pseudomonas aeruginosa* (produced by treatment with EDTA and lysozyme) restored them to an osmotically balanced state (Asbell & Eagon, 1966). The function of certain envelope components in *Achromobacter* is apparently highly dependent on divalent cations, including Ba^{2+}, and the integrity of the permeability barrier and stability of the envelope are affected at low ion concentrations (Ledebo, 1976). It has been postulated that Ba^{2+} inhibits phagocytosis of bacterial cells, thereby contributing to its cell wall stability. This has become the basis for using barium sulfate in the animal model of intra-abdominal sepsis (Bartlet et al., 1978).

7.1.3 Inhibition of growth

Growth studies have demonstrated that, in general, barium is toxic to bacteria, fungi, mosses, and algae. A low concentration of Ba^{2+} (10-100 µmol/litre) was toxic for the growth of *Nitrobacter agilis* (Tandon & Mishra, 1968). However, mutants of *Aspergillus nidulans* have been isolated that can grow in toxic concentrations of Ba^{2+} and other divalent cations. In general, the resistance of the mutants to the metal ions is the result of modified intracellular metabolism rather than defective transport (Elorza, 1969). Ba^{2+} at concentrations of 100 µmol/litre not only inhibited the growth of *Azotobacter* but also reduced slime formation and pigmentation (Dejong & Roman, 1971).

The membrane potential of the ciliate Paramecium is sensitive to intra-cellular calcium (Brehm et al., 1978). Ba^{2+}, like Ca^{2+}, spontaneously changes the membrane potential of *Paramecium caudatum*, making it resemble the long-lasting potential found in cardiac muscle fibres and smooth muscle cells. Upon replacement of calcium ions with barium ions, the normal swimming behaviour of *Paramecium multimicronucleatum* in an essential mineral solution (200 μmol Ca^{2+}/litre) changed into continuous avoidance reactions (Kinosita et al., 1964; Yarbrough & O'Kelley, 1962).

The toxic effects of Ba^{2+} and other divalent cations to Paramecium has been found to increase in alkaline and decrease in acid solutions. The effect was most noticeable at the isoelectric point of the cell surface (Grebecki & Kuznicki, 1963). The observation that an increase in Ba^{2+} concentration increased the staining of *Escherischia coli* and *Shigella ellipsoideus* with the anionic fluorochrome, uranin, supports the earlier finding (Kononenko & Chaikina, 1970).

Den Dooren de Jong (1965) reported that the highest concentration of barium tolerated by cultures of *Chlorella vulgaris* without affecting growth was 4 mg per litre and the lowest inhibitory concentration was 8 mg per litre. Problems with the precipitation of barium from the culture solution as the sulfate suggested to the author that the above results might have been artificially high. Devi Prasad (1984) found that barium inhibited calcification of the freshwater green alga Gloeotaenium at a concentration of 50 mg/litre.

7.1.4 Specific effects

The divalent barium ion has a number of specific effects, mostly toxic or inhibitory to cellular processes, on different species of bacteria and fungi. Barium inhibits the lipolytic activity of the intact cells of *Mycobacterium rubrum* and is a potent inhibitor for *Actinomyces streptomycini* (Lebedena et al., 1976). The Ba^{2+} ion has been shown to inhibit the dehydrogenase activities of resting cells of *Proteus vulgaris* (Lilov & Zahn, 1967) and to inhibit flocculation in *Saccharomyces cerevisiae* (Taylor & Orton, 1973).

The divalent barium ion may cause dissociation of the polyribosome-mRNA complex in *Paramecium aurelia* and a marked decrease in the amount of monoribosomes (Reisner et al., 1975).

The production of aflatoxins by *Aspergillus* is affected by the Ba^{2+} ion (Lee et al., 1966, Gupta et al.,

1975). Similarly, the production of α-amylase was increased by 65% in *Baccillus cereus mycoides* by barium chloride (Yoshiyuki & Yoshimasha, 1975).

The Ba^{2+} ion has been reported to affect the development of germinating bacterial spores (Rode & Foster, 1966; Foerster & Foster, 1966).

7.2 Aquatic organisms

7.2.1 Aquatic plants

Wang (1986) reported a 96-h EC_{50} of 26 mg barium per litre in *Lemma minor* in deionised water. However, in river water the barium showed no toxic effect on growth of the duckweed. Further experiments showed that the effect was entirely due to precipitation of barium from the river water as sulfate and, therefore, reduced bioavailability to the plant. Stanley (1974) investigated the toxic effect on the growth of Eurasian water milfoil *Myriophyllum spicatum*. Root weight was the most sensitive parameter measured and showed a 50% reduction, relative to controls, at a barium concentration of 41.2 mg/litre.

7.2.2 Aquatic animals

Details of studies on the lethal effects of barium salts to aquatic invertebrates and fish are given in Table 10.

LeBlanc (1980) exposed water fleas (*Daphnia magna*) in a 48-h test to various concentrations of barium and calculated the no-observed-effect level (NOEL) to be 68 mg/litre. In contrast, Biesinger & Christensen (1972) reported 48-h and 21-day LC_{50} values of 14.5 and 13.5 mg/litre, respectively. They also measured the reproductive performance of the daphnids during the 21-day tests and reported 16% impairment of reproduction at 5.8 mg barium/litre and 50% impairment at 8.9 mg/litre. In the same study, a reduction in average weight was also observed. The 30-day LC_{50} values for two species of crayfish were comparable to the 96-h values (Boutet & Chaisemartin, 1973).

Heitmuller et al. (1981) reported a no-observed-effect level in the sheepshead minnow of 500 mg/litre.

Table 10. Toxicity of barium to aquatic organisms

Organism	Lifestage/size	Stat/flow[a]	Temperature (°C)	pH	Hardness (mg/litre)	Duration	LC$_{50}$ (mg/litre)	Reference
Water flea (*Daphnia magna*) (fresh water)	<24 h old	stat	21-23	7.4-9.4	173	24 h	>530	LeBlanc (1980)
	<24 h old	stat	21-23	7.4-9.4	173	48 h	410 (320-530)	LeBlanc (1980)
				7.4-8.2	44-53	48 h	14.5	Biesinger & Christensen (1972)
				7.4-8.2	44-53	21 days	13.5[b] (12.2-15.0)	
Crayfish (*Orconectes limosus*) (fresh water)		flow	15-17	7.0		96 h	78	Boutet & Chaisemartin (1973)
		flow	15-17	7.0		30 days	59	Boutet & Chaisemartin (1973)
		flow	15-17	7.0		30 days	61[b]	Boutet & Chaisemartin (1973)
Crayfish (*Austropotamobius pallipes pallipes*) (fresh water)		flow	15-17	7.0		96 h	46	Boutet & Chaisemartin (1973)
		flow	15-17	7.0		30 days	39	Boutet & Chaisemartin (1973)
		flow	15-17	7.0		30 days	43[b]	Boutet & Chaisemartin (1973)
Sheepshead minnow (*Cyprinodon variegatus*) (marine water)	8-15 mm	stat	25-31		10-31[c]	96 h	> 500	Heitmuller et al. (1981)

[a] stat = static conditions (water unchanged for the duration of the test); flow = intermittent flow-through conditions.
[b] test conducted with a food source.
[c] salinity (°/oo).

Effects on Organisms in the Environment

7.2.3 Effects of marine drilling muds

Studies have been carried out to assess the environmental impact of offshore drilling on marine organisms. Barite (barium sulfate) is the principal constituent of drilling mud used in oil drilling operations. However, these muds contain metals other than barium. Any adverse effects on organisms not due to the physical effects of barite could be the result of the toxicity of metals other than barium.

Daugherty (1951) exposed a number of unspecified marine fish, crustaceans, and molluscs to various levels (as high as 7500 mg/kg) of drilling clay or drilling mud for an unspecified period of time. No deaths occurred and the materials were designated as non-toxic. Grantham & Sloan (1975) reported that sailfin mollies *(Poecilia latipinna)* survived a 96-h exposure to a 10% suspension of barite in both salt water and fresh water.

Togatz & Tobia (1978), and Cantelmo et al. (1979) observed the development of estuarine communities in sands mixed with (or covered by) barite. Aquaria containing specific mixtures (sand only; 1:10 barite-sand mixture; 1:3 barite-sand mixture; and sand covered by 0.5 cm of barite) were prepared in duplicate and exposed for 10 weeks to flowing estuarine water. The estuarine water naturally contained planktonic larvae. The mollusc population (individuals and species) were significantly reduced in the aquarium with the barite cover but not in the aquaria containing the barite mixtures. Annelids were reduced in all barite treatments. It was not possible to determine whether these results were due to larval avoidance of barite or to barite toxicity.

Similarly, George (1975) reported reduced biomass and diversity of fouling organisms on test panels suspended in a turbidity plume of drilling mud off the Louisiana coast, USA. However, he suggested that this result stemmed from the physical, rather than chemical, effects of the suspended material.

7.3 Bioconcentration

Marine concentrations of barium are lowest in nutrient-depleted surface waters and generally increase with depth. This suggests that barium is incorporated into organisms in the euphotic zone and is subsequently sedimented and released in deeper waters. Thus, the pattern of barium distribution in ocean waters is consistent with the conclusion of various authors that barium is actively taken up by marine organisms (Wolgemuth & Brocker, 1970; Chow, 1976; Chan et al., 1977). Wolgemuth & Brocker (1970) suggested that organisms forming opal (SiO_2) are primarily responsible for this phenomenon, but sufficient data to verify this are not available (Chan et al., 1977).

The content of barium in several types of marine algae, mollusc shells, and corals has been discussed in terms of "accumulation" or "discrimination" (Bowen, 1956). Accumulation (A[Ba]) was defined as the ratio of the barium concentration in dried tissue to that in water. Discrimination (D[Ba,Ca]) was defined as the ratio of barium to calcium in the tissue compared with the ratio of these two elements in sea water. Algae tend to accumulate barium with a large discrimination factor, whereas mollusc shells and corals accumulate somewhat higher amounts but with a relatively lower discrimination factor.

Studies by Havlik et al. (1980) using different concentrations of ^{133}Ba in algal culture media showed that barium was accumulated in algae. After 15 days exposure, the uptake by algae was 30-60% of the added amount of barium at concentrations of 0.04, 0.46, and 4.0 µg/litre medium. The lower the barium concentration in the medium, the higher was its relative accumulation in algae. The amount of barium taken up increased with the length of exposure. Barium was not incorporated into the organic components of the protoplasm but was bound primarily to the cell membrane or some other non-extractable algal components (Havlik et al., 1980).

Guthrie et al. (1979) compared the levels of barium in water and sediment from a marine area contaminated with heavy metals with the levels in various organisms. The water and sediment concentrations of barium were 7.7 mg/litre and 131.0 mg/kg wet weight, respectively. Of the organisms analysed (barnacles, crabs, oysters, clams, and polychaete worms), only barnacles showed higher concentrations of barium than that of the water (40.5 mg/kg wet weight). Stary et al. (1984) investigated the accumulation of barium ions (as ^{133}Ba) into cells of the algae *Scenedesmus obliquus* as a function of pH. Accumulation increased with increasing pH between pH 4 and 7, reaching a plateau at pH 7 and remaining constant over the range pH 7 to 9. The initial concentration of barium in the culture medium was 10^{-6} mol/litre. The K_m (affinity constant) for the accumulation of barium was calculated to be 4.8.

Barium has also been detected in the ash of Alaskan/Arctic mosses (Rastorfer, 1974).

8. EFFECTS ON EXPERIMENTAL ANIMALS AND *IN VITRO* SYSTEMS

8.1 Acute exposure

8.1.1 Oral route

The acute toxicity of various barium compounds is shown in Table 11, where doses are expressed either as LD_{50} or as the lowest lethal dose (as reported in RTECS (1985). Additional information regarding the observed non-lethal acute effects of barium is reported in Table 12.

8.1.2 Inhalation route

To assess the possible hazard of metal fumes resulting from certain metal arc-welding and other metal processing operations, Hicks et al. (1986) carried out inhalation studies in anaesthetized guinea-pigs. Collected particulate material from fumes generated by manual arc-welding (with electrodes using barium fluoride or carbonate) was extracted with dilute hydrochloric acid to give a solution containing barium. Aerosols generated from the barium fume extract were inhaled intratracheally by mechanical ventilation and were found to cause bronchoconstriction to the same extent as the inhalation of pure barium chloride (90 $\mu g/m^3$ per min).

8.1.3 Parenteral administration

In studies by Syed & Hosain (1972), the intravenous LD_{50} for barium chloride in ICR white mice was 19.2 mg barium/kg, and the values for barium nitrate and acetate were similar. These values were approximately double those reported for Swiss-Webster mice.

Roza & Berman (1971) found that barium chloride infused intravenously into anaesthetized dogs caused ectopic ventricular contractions, skeletal muscle paralysis, salivation, and, finally, respiratory paralysis and ventricular fibrillation. These effects were due to a prompt and substantial hypokalaemia and could be prevented or

Table 11. Acute toxicity of various barium compounds in laboratory animals[a]

Compound	Species	Route	Dose[b] (mg/kg body weight)		
Barium acetate	ICR mouse	iv	LD_{50}	=	23.3[c]
Barium carbonate	rat	oral	LD_{50}	=	418
	rat	oral	LD_{50}	=	800[d]
	mouse	iv	LLD	=	20
	mouse	oral	LD_{50}	=	200
	mouse	ip	LD_{50}	=	50
	dog	oral	LLD	=	400
Barium chloride	rat	oral	LD_{50}	=	118
	rat	sc	LD_{50}	=	178
	rat	iv	LLD	=	20
	mouse	oral	LLD	=	70
	mouse	ip	LD_{50}	=	54
	mouse	sc	LLD	=	10
	mouse	iv	LD_{50}	=	12
	ICR mouse	iv	LD_{50}	=	19.2[c]
	dog	oral	LLD	=	90
	rabbit	oral	LLD	=	170
	rabbit	sc	LLD	=	55
	guinea-pig	oral	LLD	=	76
	guinea-pig	sc	LLD	=	55
	frog	sc	LLD	=	910
Barium fluoborate	rat	oral	LLD	=	250
Barium fluoride	rat	oral	LD_{50}	=	250
	mouse	ip	LD_{50}	=	29.9
	frog	sc	LLD	=	1540
Barium nitrate	rat	oral	LD_{50}	=	355
	mouse	sc	LLD	=	10
	mouse	iv	LD_{50}	=	8.5
	ICR mouse	iv	LD_{50}	=	20.1[c]
Barium oxide	mouse	sc	LD_{50}	=	50
Barium peroxide	mouse	sc	LD_{50}	=	50
Barium polysulfide	rat	oral	LD_{50}	=	375
Barium silicofluoride	rat	oral	LD_{50}	=	175
Barium sulfide	rat	oral	LD_{50}	=	640
Barium sulfonates	rat	oral	LD_{50}	=	3000

Table 11 (contd).

Compound	Species	Route	Dose[b] (mg/kg body weight)
Barium zirconium oxide	rat	oral	LD_{50} = 1980
	rat	ip	LD_{50} = 420

[a] Source: RTECS (1985) except where stated otherwise.
[b] LLD = Lowest lethal dose: the lowest dose (other than LD_{50}) of a substance introduced by any route (except inhalation), over any given period of time in one or more divided portions, which has caused death in human beings or animals (RTECS, 1985).
[c] Source: Syed & Hosain (1972); the concentrations given are those of the Ba^{2+} ion.
[d] Source: Windholz (1983).

reversed by potassium administration. This barium-induced hypokalaemia was probably not due to potassium losses in the gastrointestinal tract or urine. The authors suggested that potassium accumulated in the intracellular compartment, since the red blood cell potassium level was elevated by barium chloride infusion.

Topical route

In rabbits, barium nitrate causes mild skin irritation (24-h exposure) and severe eye irritation (24-h exposure) (RTECS, 1985).

Short-term exposures

Inhalation route

The effects of short-term exposure to barium compounds in animals are summarized in Table 12. Tarasenko et al. (1977) carried out a series of subchronic experiments with rats to measure the effects of inhalation exposure to barium (as barium carbonate dust). Male rats exposed to barium carbonate at concentrations of 1.15 and 5.2 mg/m^3 for 4 months, 6 days/week, 4 h/day, experienced decreased weight gain, blood sugar, and haemoglobin, as well as leucocytosis and thrombopenia in the high-dose group. Increase in arterial pressure was also noted. No adverse effects were reported in the low-dose group. In a second study, male rats exposed to barium carbonate (22.6 mg/m^3)

Table 12. Effects of acute and chronic exposure to barium compounds in experimental animals

Compound	Species	Concentration	Route	Duration	Observation	Reference
Barium chloride	rat	1, 10, 100 mg/litre	oral (water)	16 months	depressed cardiac rates and excitability; decreased cardiac ATP, phosphocreatine, and phosphorylation potential	Perry et al. (1985)
	rat	1, 10, 100 mg/litre	oral (water)	16 months	Increased systolic pressure, decreased conductivity and conduction	Perry et al. (1985)
	rat	100 mg/litre	oral (water)	16 months	induced disturbances of myocardial contractility, hypersensitivity to phenobarbital and shortening cardiac muscle fibre velocity	Kopp et al. (1985)
	mouse	2, 6.6, 20 mg/kg	ip		CNS effects; convulsive corneal electroshock; sensitivity increased after 0.5 h; decrease in electroshock sensitivity at 24 h	Peyton & Borowitz (1978)
	pig	1.7 mg/kg per min	iv infusion	20 min	cardiovascular toxicity; bradycardia	Pento (1979)
	dog	0.5-2.0 μmol/kg per min	iv infusion	10-100 min	stimulation of cardiac, smooth, and skeletal muscles manifested by arrhythmia, diarrhoea, and skeletal muscle twitching; hypokalaemia, hypertension, direct stimulation of arterial smooth muscle	Roza & Berman (1971)
	dog	initial: 3.6-64.7 μmol/kg per min; thereafter: 0.5-1.0 μmol/kg per min	iv infusion	2-10 min	accelerated ventricular escapes; tachycardia	Foster et al. (1977)

Table 12. (contd).

Barium carbonate	rat and rabbit	33.4 mg/m^3	inhalation		hematopoietic differences; reduction in detoxifying function in liver; desquamative bronchitis	Tarasenko et al. (1977)
	rat	5.2 mg/m^3	inhalation	4 h/day 6 days/week 4 months	pronounced general toxic effect and influence on mineral metabolism and PNS	Tarasenko et al. (1977)
	rat	22.6 mg/m^3	inhalation	not stated	disturbance of spermatogenesis; fewer viable sperm cells	Tarasenko et al. (1977)
	rat	5.2 mg/m^3	inhalation	4 months	disturbance of spermatogenesis	Tarasenko et al. (1977)
	rat	3.1 and 13.4 mg/m^3	inhalation	4 months	disturbance of oestrous cycle and ovary morphology	Tarasenko et al. (1977)
	rat	26 mg/kg	oral	29 days before conception and during entire pregnancy	increased mortality of offspring; embryotoxic effects	Tarasenko et al. (1977)
Barium acetate	rat	5 mg/litre (water)	oral	540 days	slightly increased mortality in females; increase in growth after 150 days over controls	Schroeder & Mitchener (1975a)
	mouse	5 mg/litre (water)	oral	540 days	longevity slightly reduced in males, but weight not significantly affected; no change in prevalence of tumours, oedema, or blanching of incisor teeth	Schroeder & Mitchener (1975b)

Effects on Experimental Animals and In Vitro Systems

for one cycle of spermatogenesis showed a decrease in spermatozoids, sperm motility, and osmotic resistance. There was also a significant increase in the number of ducts with desquamative epithelium and a reduction in the number of ducts with 12th-stage meiosis. The authors indicated that similar spermatogenic changes were observed in male rats exposed for 4 months at 5.2 mg/m^3.

Inhalation exposure of female rats to barium carbonate (3.1 or 13.4 mg/m^3) produced a shortening of the oestrous cycle and changes in ovary morphology. In addition, females exposed to 13.4 mg/m^3 had increased mortality and underdeveloped offspring (Tarasenko et al., 1977).

8.2.2 Oral route

To assess adverse effects resulting from exposure to high levels of barium in drinking-water, Borzelleca et al. (1988) administered, by gavage, barium chloride (30, 100, or 300 mg/kg body weight for 1 day or 100, 145, 209, or 300 mg/kg body weight for 10 days) to male and female Sprague-Dawley rats. In the 1-day exposure study, decreases in body weight and liver/brain weight ratios and an increase in kidney weight were found at 300 mg/kg. In animals exposed for 10 days, there was a decrease in the survival rate of females given 300 mg/kg. Reductions in ovary/brain ratios and blood urea nitrogen (BUN) levels were also reported for females. In males, the BUN levels were decreased at 300 mg/kg. No other effects were reported.

In studies by Tardiff et al. (1980), barium chloride was added to tap water at concentrations of 0, 10, 50, and 250 mg barium/litre and fed to 4-week-old Charles River rats (30 of each sex per group). A commercial diet containing an average barium concentration of 6.6 ± 0.5 µg/kg was given, approximating to a background daily dose of 0.5 µg barium/kg body weight. At 4, 8, and 13 weeks of exposure, five rats of each sex from each dosage level were killed, biochemical and haematological parameters were measured, and histopathological examinations were performed. No clinical signs of toxicity were manifested during the exposure to barium chloride. Throughout the duration of the study, the body weights of treated animals were similar to the control values. No statistically significant differences between exposed and control animals were observed for any of the haematological or biochemical parameters measured; values for all animals were within normal limits during the course of the study. No gross or microscopic abnormalities were found in the liver, kidneys, spleen, heart, brain, muscle, femur, or adrenals. The relative weight of adrenals in male rats treated for 8 (but not 13) weeks at 50 and 250 mg/litre decreased significantly. The relative weight of adrenals in female rats after 13 weeks of exposure to 10, 50, or 250 mg/litre was slightly decreased. The effect did not appear to be dose- or duration-related in either sex.

In a series of studies, McCauley et al. (1985) investigated the histological and cardiovascular effects on rats exposed to barium chloride in drinking water. Male Sprague-Dawley rats (6 per group) were exposed to 0, 1, 10, 100, or 250 mg barium/litre in their drinking-water for 36 weeks or to 0, 1, 10, 100, or 1000 mg/litre for 16 weeks. No histopathological abnormalities were observed in any of the tissues examined. There were no significant trends toward hypertension in any of the animals treated with 100 mg/litre. Transient changes in blood pressure were reported, but these were not considered to be dose- or duration-related. Similarly, no significant histological or cardiovascular effects were observed in female Sprague-Dawley rats exposed to 0 or 250 mg barium/litre for 46 weeks. However, animals receiving 1000 mg barium per litre did exhibit ultrastructural changes in the kidney glomeruli, including basement membrane thickening, epithelial foot process fusion, and the presence of myelin figures. No other effects were reported at any dose levels for males or females.

8.3 Long-term exposure

8.3.1 Inhalation route

No pertinent data regarding chronic inhalation exposure to barium have been found in the available literature.

8.3.2 Oral route

The effects of chronic exposure to barium compounds in experimental animals are summarized in Table 12. McCauley et al. (1985) studied the effects on male Sprague-Dawley rats of exposure to drinking-water containing 0, 10, 100, or 250 mg barium per litre for 68 weeks. Rats exposed to 250 mg/litre for 5 months were then challenged with an arrhythmagenic dose of L-noradrenaline (5 µg/kg iv). Barium-treated animals demonstrated no significant histological changes in 34 tissue types examined, and no changes in body weight or food and water consumption were reported. No increase in the incidence of tumours was reported. All tumours were benign and uniformly distributed. The rats challenged with L-noradrenaline demonstrated no significant ECG changes when compared to controls. However, the heart rate of treated animals was significantly lower 4 min after the injection, but returned to normal within 60 min.

Schroeder & Mitchener (1975a) studied the effects of lifetime exposure to barium acetate (0 or 5 mg/litre) in the drinking-water and low-trace-element diets of weanling Long-Evans rats (52 of each sex). Animals were weighed at weekly intervals initially, monthly for 1 year, and finally at 3-month intervals. Barium had no significant effect on the growth of males, but significantly increased growth rates were seen in females aged 120 days in 4 of the 16 measurements. Proteinuria was observed in barium-exposed males to a greater extent than it was in the controls. No differences were found in serum glucose, cholesterol, or uric acid concentrations between exposed rats and controls.

Using the same exposure details, Schroeder & Mitchener (1975b) conducted a second lifetime study on Swiss mice (42 males, 36 females). No effects were observed on growth rate or body weight except in the case of female mice who weighed slightly less than controls at 30 days. At 60 days, there was no difference between the weights of control and treated mice. No effects on gross pathology or histopathology were observed. Longevity (defined as the mean age at death of the last surviving 10% of animals) was slightly reduced ($P < 0.025$) in treated males (815 days versus 920 for controls), but the average age at death did not differ (548 days, treated mice; 540 days, control mice).

Perry et al. (1983, 1985) maintained female weanling Long-Evans rats in a "low contamination" environment on a control diet low in trace metals for 16 months. Drinking-water was deionized and fortified with five essential trace metals, and 0, 1, 10, or 100 mg barium per litre (as barium chloride) was added. Based on water consumption data, average daily doses of 0.051, 0.51, and 5.1 mg/kg were calculated. Barium produced no change in growth rate, and no evidence of toxicity was detected. The indirect systolic pressure of unanaesthetized rats was measured in triplicate at 1, 2, 4, 8, 12, and 16 months (Perry et al., 1983, 1985). The average systolic pressure was significantly increased ($P < 0.001$) after exposure to 100 mg barium/litre for 1 month, and after exposure to 10 mg/litre ($P < 0.025$) for 8 months. Average increases at 1, 12, and 16 months for the highest dose were 1.6, 2.13, and 2.13 kPa (12, 16, and 16 mmHg), respectively. With the 10-mg/litre dose, increases of 0.8, 0.93, and 0.53 kPa (6, 7, and 4 mmHg) were observed at 8, 12, and 16 months, respectively. At the highest dose there was a decrease at 16 months in cardiac ATP, phosphocreatine, and phosphorylation potential, and an increase in ADP levels. Kopp et al. (1985) analysed the *in vivo* myocardial excitability, contractility, and metabolic characteristics of the highest-dose rats at 16 months and observed significant barium-induced disturbances in myocardial contractility. The most distinctive effect demonstrated was a hypersensitivity of the cardiovascular system to sodium pentobarbital. Under barbiturate anaesthesia, virtually all of the myocardial contractile indices were depressed significantly in barium-exposed rats. The lack of a similar response to ketamine and xylazine anaesthesia indicated that the cardiovascular actions of sodium pentobarbital in barium-treated rats were linked specifically to this anaesthetic and were not representative of a generalized anaesthetic response. The contractile element shortening velocity of the cardiac muscle fibres was significantly slower in barium-treated rats relative to the control rats. Similarly, significant disturbances in myocardial energy metabolism were detected in the barium-exposed rats. These disturbances were consistent with the reduced contractile element shortening velocity. In addition, the excitability of the cardiac conduction system was depressed preferentially in the atrioventricular nodal region of hearts from barium-exposed rats. Overall, the altered cardiac contractility and excitability characteristics, the myocardial metabolic disturbances, and the hypersensitivity of the cardiovascular system to the sodium pentobarbital suggest the existence of a previously undescribed cardiomyopathic disorder induced by chronic barium exposure.

8.4 Reproduction, embryotoxicity, and teratogenicity

8.4.1 Reproduction

Inhalation exposure of male rats to barium carbonate (22.6 mg/m^3 for one spermatogenic cycle or 5.2 mg/m^3 for 4 months) resulted in a decrease in spermatozoids and a reduction in the number of ducts with 12th stage necrosis. Females exposed to barium carbonate (3.1 or 13.4 mg/m^3) experienced a shortening of the oestrous cycle and increased mortality, and their pups were underdeveloped (Silayev & Tarasenko, 1976; Tarasenko et al., 1977). Other reproductive effects observed for various barium compounds, as reported in RTECS (1985), are listed in Table 13.

8.4.2 Embryotoxicity and teratogenicity

Barium fluoride orally administered (at 0.03-0.1 of the LD_{50} value) to rats on the first days of gestation decreased the percentage of 5-day-old embryos in the blastomeric stage and newborn birth weights (Popova & Peretolcyina, 1976). In addition, the death rate in newborn rats was higher than normal. No teratogenic effects were reported. Since fluoride inhibits many biochemical processes, the results may reflect the presence of fluoride rather than barium. Tarasenko et al. (1977) exposed rats to barium carbonate (3.1 and 13.4 mg/m^3), for 24 days before conception and during gestation, and observed an increase in the mortality of the fetuses and low birth weights but no teratogenesis.

Ridgeway & Karnofsky (1952) examined the teratogenicity of barium by injecting 20 mg barium chloride into the yolk sac of developing chick embryos. When the injection was made on day 8 of development, developmental

Table 13. Reproductive effects of barium compounds[a]

Compound	Route	Species	Sex	Exposure data	Effects on
Barium carbonate	inhalation	rat	male	1.15 mg/m^3 per 24 h for 16 weeks prior to mating; lowest toxic dose	spermatogenesis; testes, epididymis, sperm duct
Barium carbonate	inhalation	rat	female	3.13 mg/m^3 per 24 h for 16 weeks prior to mating; lowest toxic dose	oogenesis; ovaries, fallopian tubes
Barium iron oxide	inhalation	rat	male	0.76 mg/m^3 per 24 h for 17 weeks prior to mating; lowest toxic concentration	spermatogenesis
Barium chloride	intratracheal	rat	male	16.7 mg/kg 1 day prior to mating; lowest toxic dose	testes, epididymis, sperm duct

[a] Source: RTECS (1985).

Effects on Experimental Animals and In Vitro Systems

defects were observed in the toes. In contrast, no effects were seen when the injection was made on day 4 of development.

8.5 Mutagenicity and related end-points

Nishioka (1975) reported that barium chloride produced no increase in the mutation frequency in repair-deficient strains of *Bacillus subtilis*. Using synthetic polynucleotide templates and purified DNA polymerases, Ba^{2+} was found to have no effect on DNA synthesis, although other metals such as Cd^{2+}, Co^{2+}, Ni^{2+}, and Pb^{2+} did decrease the fidelity of DNA synthesis and were categorized as potential mutagens (Sirover & Loeb, 1976a,b).

8.6 Tumorigenicity and carcinogenicity

Schroeder & Mitchener (1975a,b) examined the long-term effects of barium and several other metals on rats and mice. Groups of Long-Evans rats (52 of each sex) and CD mice (54 of each sex) were given 0 or 5 mg barium/litre in their drinking-water throughout their life. The incidence of tumours in treated animals was not significantly different to that of control animals. It was concluded that under these conditions barium was not carcinogenic.

Barium chromate has been evaluated in monographs on chromium and chromium compounds (IARC, 1973; IARC, 1980; IARC, 1987). Barium chromate has been tested for carcinogenicity in rats by intrabronchial, intramuscular, and intrapleural administration. No lung tumours were produced after intrabronchial implantation, but the other experiments were considered inadequate to evaluate carcinogenicity. IARC considered that there is sufficient evidence for the carcinogenicity of hexavalent chromium compounds in animals and humans (Group 1: carcinogenic to humans). This evaluation applied to the group of chemicals as a whole and not necessarily to each individual chemical within the group (IARC, 1987).

8.7 Special studies

8.7.1 *Effects on the heart*

The studies of Slavicek (1972), Katzung & Morgenstern (1976), Foster et al. (1977), Meier & Katzung (1978),

Shine et al. (1978), and Pento (1979) have presented evidence of the detrimental effect of barium on ventricular automacity and the pacemaker current in the heart.

Infusion of barium chloride into anaesthetized dogs produced premature ventricular contractions or ventricular tachycardia (Roza & Berman, 1971). These effects were accompanied by hypokalaemia, and the administration of potassium prevented or reversed the arrhythmias. However, the increased blood pressure also associated with barium infusion was not blocked by potassium administration. Kidney removal or the administration of phentolamine, a blocking agent of α-catecholamine receptors, did not reverse the hypertension. Presumably, barium acts directly on vascular smooth muscle to cause hypertension.

More recent studies by Perry et al. (1983, 1985), Kopp et al. (1985), and Hirano & Hiraoka (1986) have shown that barium decreases cardiac contractility and excitability, and produces automaticity of ventricular muscles in rats and guinea-pigs. Barium chloride (2 mmol/litre) induced slow diastolic dipolarization and reduced membrane potential in the right ventricle of guinea-pigs (Hirano & Hiraoka, 1986).

8.7.2 Vascular effects

Using spirally cut strips of rabbit thoracic aorta suspended in a physiological test-chamber, Perry et al. (1967) tested responsiveness to various concentrations of barium ions. A slow, steady contraction was induced, which averaged 5% at 10^{-4} mol/litre and increased to 26% at 10^{-3} mol/litre.

Using intra-arterial barium chloride, Perry & Yunice (1965) demonstrated a pressure response in Sprague-Dawley rats. Barium-injected rats (6 per group) showed an average increase of 0.27 kPa (2 mmHg) in diastolic pressure after the administration of 0.1 mg Ba^{2+}/kg body weight. After 10 min, 1 mg Ba^{2+}/kg body weight was injected. Ten minutes later, an additional 10 mg Ba/kg body weight was injected. Diastolic pressure increased by 3.2 kPa (24 mmHg) ($P < 0.01$) with the 1 mg/kg injection, and by 7.47 kPa (56 mmHg) ($P < 0.01$) with the 10 mg/kg injection.

8.7.3 Electrophysiological effects

Experimental evidence indicates that barium can partially mimic calcium in many physiological processes. Studies by Silinsky (1978) and Erdelyi (1977) examined the effect of barium on nerve impulse transmission. Acetylcholine is a transmitter of nerve impulses and its release is controlled by calcium ions. When barium replaces the calcium, release of acetylcholine is stimulated, causing depolarization of the post-synaptic nerve. The barium-stimulated *in vitro* release of acetylcholine does not appear to have a feedback control mechanism similar to that involved in calcium regulation, and within 24 h the acetylcholine pool is depleted. Although barium releases acetylcholine quanta, it cannot synchronize the release with the impulsive event. Thus, despite its efficiency in supporting neurosecretion, barium is unsuitable as a normal physiological mediator of depolarization-secretion coupling at the motor nerve end (McLachlan, 1977).

An important biological action of barium is the blockade of potassium efflux from cells. The addition of barium (0.8 mmol/litre) to cell medium resulted in an increase in the release of noradrenalin from cat spleen tissue (Kirpekar et al., 1972). Hausler & Haefely (1979) have shown that when potassium efflux is blocked by barium, depolarization is prolonged. This allows for greater cellular influx of calcium during depolarization and accounts for the enhanced effect of nerve stimulation in the presence of barium (Hausler & Haefely, 1979).

Barium can also affect calcium metabolism by blocking its efflux from cells. Concentrations of 0.3 mmol/litre inhibited by 41% the ATPase-mediated extrusion of calcium in bovine adrenomedullary plasma membrane preparations (Leslie & Borowitz, 1975). Owing to its ability to block calcium efflux from cells, barium may have widespread effects in secretory tissues and, possibly, in certain muscle tissues. In frog sartorious muscle, barium (0.01 mmol/litre) inhibited potassium uptake and efflux symmetrically (Henderson & Volle, 1972).

Pappano (1976) studied the electrophysiological action of barium in chick embryo atria and compared it to that of calcium. The ability of barium to evoke an action potential decreased during ontogeny, but barium was more potent than calcium in generating an action potential. Based on these findings, the author suggested that barium can enter the cell by the same mechanism as calcium.

8.7.4 Effects on synaptic transmission and catecholamine release

Calcium is an essential ion in a number of secretory processes, especially in the release of neurotransmitters (Rubin, 1970). Barium mimics this action and can evoke the release of (1) acetylcholine from the neuromuscular junction (Silinsky, 1978), (2) acetylcholine from the sympathetic ganglia (McLachan, 1977), (3) noradrenaline from the sympathetic nerve terminals (Rubin, 1970), and (4) catecholamines from the adrenal medulla (Douglas & Rubin, 1964a,b; Shanbaky et al., 1978).

The mode of release of neurotransmitter by barium is distinct from that by calcium. Calcium can evoke the release of neurotransmitter only when the nerve membranes are depolarized by nerve impulse. On the other hand, barium can evoke the release of transmitter without previous depolarization. Another characteristic of the barium-evoked release is that it is persistent, while release by calcium is transitory and terminated by membrane repolarization.

The action of barium in triggering the release of catecholamine was examined in detail using cultured bovine chromaffin cells. Heldman et al. (1989) showed that barium can enter cells via the voltage-dependent Ca-channels without previous depolarization. Izumi et al. (1986) showed that micromolar concentrations of barium can evoke the secretion of catecholamines after removal of calcium by a calcium chelating agent. This suggests that barium can trigger the secretory process by itself, not merely via the cellular calcium.

8.7.5 Effects on the immune system

According to Kolpakov (1971), immune mechanisms may be influenced by barium. Rats given barium chloride every other day for 3-4 weeks showed marked leucocytosis. An iv injection of 1.5-2.0 ml of blood serum from barium-treated rats into untreated rats caused a marked increase in leucocytosis. Barium chloride may have enhanced the production of leucopoeitins.

Mouse peritoneal macrophages exposed to barium sulfate for up to 144 h showed marked cytoplasmic vacuolization with only partial recovery (Rae, 1977).

8.7.6 Ocular system

Studies by Sowden & Pirie (1958) indicated that barium may play a role in normal vision. Using neutron-activation analysis, the pigmented parts of eyeballs were found to contain a higher barium content than the other parts. Although the precise function of the metal is unknown, it was suggested that the presence of barium might be essential for the function and structure of the choroid and for vision. This may be the only biological role ascribable to barium.

9. EFFECTS ON MAN

9.1 General population exposure

9.1.1 Acute toxicity - poisoning incidents

There have been several reports of barium poisoning due to ingestion of barium chloride (Graham, 1934; Allen, 1943, Wang et al., 1989) or barium carbonate (Morton, 1945; Lewi & Bar-Khayim, 1964; Diengott et al., 1964; Phelan et al., 1984) or due to the diagnostic use of barium sulfate in gastrointestinal tract studies (Gray et al., 1989; Ahmed & Hamza, 1989; Feczko et al., 1989).

It has been estimated that the lethal dose of barium in untreated cases is 3-4 g (66 mg/kg body weight) and the threshold for a toxic dose is 0.2-0.5 g (Reeves, 1986). These values apply to the portion absorbed from the gut. A lethal dose for barium chloride of 11.4 mg/kg has been reported in RTECS (1985) (Table 14). Barium carbonate and barium sulfide are also toxic, but act more slowly (Sollman, 1953).

Table 14. Toxicity of barium compounds to humans[a]

Compound	Exposure data	Effect
Barium carbonate	lowest lethal dose = 57 mg/kg	death
Barium carbonate	lowest toxic dose = 29 mg/kg	flaccid paralysis without anaesthesia; paraesthesia; muscle weakness
Barium chloride	lowest lethal dose = 11.4 mg/kg	death
Barium polysulfide	lowest toxic dose = 226 mg/kg	flaccid paralysis without anaesthesia; muscle weakness; dyspnoea

[a] Source: RTECS (1985).

Several hundred cases of acute or subacute barium poisoning occurred in the Kiating district of China, where table salt contained a large amount of barium (up to 26%). The victims suffered sudden attacks of paralysis, ranging from mild to severe, paraesthesia, and cardiac symptoms, but recovery was usually rapid (Allen, 1943).

Another instance of barium poisoning affected over a hundred people who had all consumed sausages made with barium carbonate instead of potato meal (Lewi & Bar-Khayim, 1964). Of the large number of people affected only 19 were hospitalized. Symptoms ranged from mild vomiting and diarrhoea to partial paralysis.

Diengott et al. (1964) reported two further cases of food poisoning resulting from the ingestion of the contaminated sausage. In both cases, the patients experienced severe weakness, diarrhoea, and paralysis. One patient died suddenly after developing right facial paralysis and left hemiplegia. The second patient recovered.

Four recent cases of fatal barium poisoning and hypersensitivity have been reported by Ahmed & Hamza, (1989), Gray et al. (1989), and Feczko et al. (1989). In two of the cases, death was the result of acute hypersensitivity reaction following treatment with radioactive barium sulfate contrast medium. The remaining two deaths resulted from acute inflammation of the bronchi and peripheral airways after accidental inhalation of barium sulfate.

In a reported case of an attempted suicide, the ingestion of 40 g barium carbonate resulted in a plasma potassium level of 1.5 mmol/litre (approximately one third the normal serum potassium level) and induced muscle weakness, respiratory failure, and complete paralysis. Normal muscular and renal function was regained within 7 days (Phelan et al., 1984).

The rapid onset of reflex paralysis was reported in a chrome-plating worker following the inhalation of barium powder. Complete recovery occurred during the 5-day period that followed exposure (Shankle & Keane, 1988). Wang et al. (1989) reported two cases of barium poisoning resulting from scalding with barium chloride solution. In both instances cardiac dysfunction was reported and one patient died due to sudden cardiac arrest.

There are three stages of barium poisoning: a) acute gastroenteritis; b) loss of deep reflexes with onset of muscular paralysis; and c) progressive muscular paralysis. The muscular paralysis seems to be related to severe hypokalaemia. These three stages need not be present in each patient for barium poisoning to be suspected. In most cases, recovery is rapid and uneventful. Treatment generally consists of intravenous infusion of potassium carbonate or lactate and/or oral administration of sodium sulfate to precipitate the barium as barium sulfate (Centro de Informacion Toxicologica, 1972).

Potassium infusion has been used clinically to reverse the toxic effects of barium. A patient who attempted suicide by ingesting a commercial depilatory containing barium sulfide (12.8 g barium were ingested) showed marked skeletal muscle paralysis and required assisted respiration. Potassium was infused intravenously as an antidote and full recovery was achieved within 24 h (Gould et al., 1973).

9.1.2 Short-term controlled human studies

Wones et al. (1990) administered barium (as barium chloride) in the drinking-water of 11 healthy male volunteers at levels found in the drinking water of some communities in the USA. Subjects ranged in age from 27 to 61 years and had no previous history of diabetes, hypertension, or cardiovascular disease of any kind. Diets were strictly controlled throughout the 10-week study. Subjects were given 1.5 litres/day of distilled and charcoal-filtered water containing no barium for the first 2 weeks, 5 mg/litre for weeks 3-6, and 10 mg/litre for weeks 7-10. Blood and urine samples as well as morning and evening blood pressures were measured throughout the study. In addition, electrocardiograms and 24-h continuous electrocardiographic monitoring were performed for 2 consecutive days at the end of each study period. No change was reported in blood pressure, total cholesterol, triglycerides, high-density lipoprotein, or low-density lipoprotein cholesterol levels. Serum potassium and glucose levels, as well as urinary metanephrine (catecholamine breakdown product) levels, were also unchanged. No significant arrhythmias were noted during the barium exposure period.

Effects on Man

There was, however, an increase in the number of premature atrial contractions, but this increase was neither statistically nor clinically significant. There was a slight increase in total serum calcium levels. Blood protein levels were unchanged. Although this study was limited by its small sample size and the brief duration of exposure, the authors concluded that drinking-water levels of 5 and 10 mg/litre barium did not have a significant impact on the cardiovascular system.

9.1.3 Epidemiological studies

9.1.3.1 Cardiovascular disease

In two limited epidemiological studies, the negative correlation between barium levels in drinking-water and cardiovascular mortalities was questionable (Elwood et al., 1974, and Schroeder & Kraemer, 1974).

Brenniman et al. (1979) conducted a retrospective study, for the years 1971-1975, of the association between age- and sex-adjusted cardiovascular death rates and barium levels in the drinking-water in 16 Illinois (USA) communities. Comparisons of these death rates were made between communities that had high barium levels in their public drinking-water supplies (2.0-10 mg/litre) and communities with low barium levels (<0.2 mg/litre). Study communities were matched for population, ethnic characteristics, age distribution, number of persons per household, number of school years completed, and mean income. The study showed a high correlation between age-adjusted death rates from all cardiovascular disease and areas with high barium levels. However, some of the communities that had high barium levels also had a 70% change in their population between 1960 and 1970. Additionally, there was no method of controlling removal of barium by home water-softeners. For these reasons, the finding of an association between barium level and death due to "all cardiovascular disease" and "heart disease" must be interpreted with caution. Increased death rates caused by hypertension were examined, as suggested by Calabrese (1977), and no correlation was found.

As a follow-up to their earlier study, Brenniman et al. (1981) conducted a cross-sectional study, for the years 1976-1977, of the association between intake of elevated barium levels in drinking-water and elevated blood pressure. One community that had high barium levels (West Dundee, Illinois, mean barium level of 7.3 mg/litre) and one community that had low barium (McHenry, Illinois, mean barium level of 0.1 mg/litre) were studied. All other drinking-water constituents were nearly identical between the two communities. In a questionnaire answered by the participants in this study, information was obtained on the following variables: age, sex, weight, height, smoking habits, family history of disease, occupation, and medication (with special reference to blood pressure medication). In addition, information was obtained on the length of residence in the community and the frequency of use of a water-softener or other home water-treatment device.

No significant differences in blood pressure were found between the populations that had high and low barium intakes. These findings were not altered by adjustment for home water-softener use, duration of exposure, or medication for high blood pressure. In addition to these findings, no differences, with respect to heart disease, stroke, or kidney disease, were found between the commununities that had high barium levels in drinking-water and those with low levels. It was concluded that high levels of barium in drinking-water do not significantly elevate blood pressure levels in adult males or females.

9.1.3.2 *Other effects*

The possible correlation between the level of barium in the drinking-water and human congenital malformations was discussed in two studies. No association was found by Schroeder & Kraemer (1974). Morton et al. (1976), using the methodology of Elwood et al. (1974), found a negative association between the concentration of barium in the drinking-water and the presence of malformations in the central nervous system. However, the data do not allow any firm conclusions to be drawn.

The prevalence of dental caries was reported to be significantly lower in 39 children residing in a community supplied with drinking-water containing high barium concentrations (8-10 mg/litre) than in 36 children from a

Effects on Man

similar community with drinking-water concentrations of <3.0 mg/litre (Zdanowicz et al., 1987).

9.2 Occupational exposure

9.2.1 Effects of short- and long-term exposure

It has been known for many years that workers exposed to finely ground barium salts develop baritosis consisting of a mixture of very fine punctate and annular lesions and some slightly larger nodular lesions (Pendergrass & Greening, 1953). Pronin & Pashkovskii (1973) reported that cardiac activity disturbances noted in 31 out of 60 workers exposed to barium salts for 3-22 years possibly reflect the effect of barium on cell potassium levels. These studies suggest that the heart may be a primary target for the action of barium in humans. Workers at a barite factory were monitored for lung deposition of barium (Doig, 1976). Chest radiographs showed dense shadows, which slowly disappeared when exposure to barite ceased. Affected workers showed no symptoms, no abnormal physical signs, no loss of vital capacity, no interference with lung function, and no evidence of increased susceptibility to pulmonary infections. NIOSH (1982) conducted an environmental and medical investigation at a mineral processing plant. Barium workers had a significantly higher incidence of hypertension than did non-barium workers (58% versus 20%). Barium exposure resulting from the grinding and mixing of several grades of barium-containing ore ("baryte process") ranged from 0.8 to 1.92 mg/m^3, with a mean of 1.07 mg/m^3

Recently, four cases of pneumoconiosis were reported in barium miners in Scotland (Seaton et al., 1986). Of the miners who had developed pneumoconiosis, three developed progressive massive fibrosis, from which two died, and one developed a nodular simple pneumoconiosis after leaving the industry. The radiological and pathological features of the men's lungs were those of silicosis, which was confirmed by the high proportions of quartz that were found. There was a complete absence of barium in the lungs, suggesting that much of the barium that is inhaled is not taken into the pulmonary tissues, but remains in alveolar macrophages and is eventually removed by the mucociliary mechanism.

NIOSH (1979) investigated the environmental exposures and health status of workers and residents in the vicinity of a New York landfill. The investigation included a historical and qualitative environmental evaluation, measurements of occupational exposures to hazardous substances at three industries near the landfill, and a cross-sectional medical study of 428 people. In comparison with the data from the Health and Nutrition Examination Survey of 1971-1973, participants in the NIOSH study had higher prevalences of musculoskelatal symptoms, gastrointestinal surgery, skin problems, and respiratory symptoms. The latter was accounted for mainly by workers in the metal alloy manufacturing industry, where excessive occupational exposures were found for soluble barium (0.02-1.7 mg/m^3). However, other agents (inorganic lead, zirconium, total particulates, and UV-visible-IR radiation) were also present.

9.3 Carcinogenicity of barium chromate

Barium chromate (VI) is the only barium compound for which there is sufficient evidence that it is a human carcinogen (IARC, 1980).

IARC (1987) concluded that there is sufficient evidence for the carcinogenicity of hexavalent chromium compounds to animals and humans (Group I: carcinogenic to humans). This evaluation applied to the group of compounds as a whole and not necessarily to each individual chemical within the group.

10. EVALUATION OF HUMAN HEALTH RISKS AND EFFECTS ON THE ENVIRONMENT

10.1 Evaluation of human health risks

10.1.1 *Exposure levels*

10.1.1.1 General population

The dietary intake of barium, based on data from the USA, ranges from 300 to 1700 µg/day. The average values reported by two different sources were 600 and 900 µg/day.

Recent studies from the USA indicate barium levels in drinking-water ranging from 1 to 20 µg/litre. Based on this range and assuming a daily consumption of 2 litres of drinking-water, the intake of barium in drinking-water would be 2-40 µg/day.

The intake via inhalation is estimated to range from 0.04 to 3.1 µg/day.

The estimated total daily intake of barium in Wales (United Kingdom) is 1327 µg (food 1240 µg; drinking-water 86 µg; air 1 µg).

10.1.1.2 Occupational - air exposures

Exposure of metal alloy workers to concentrations ranging from 0.08 to 1.92 mg/m^3 (mean: 1.07 mg/m^3) resulted in a high prevalence of hypertension. In a group of mineral ore processors experiencing musculoskeletal and respiratory symptoms, barium exposures of 0.02 to 1.7 mg/m^3 were reported. Exposures of steel arc welders to concentrations ranging from 2.2 to 6.1 mg/m^3 have been measured. These are the highest occupational levels that have been reported, but no medical studies were conducted.

10.1.1.3 Acute exposures

Barium doses as low as 0.2-0.5 g (3-7 mg/kg body weight), generally resulting from the ingestion of barium chloride or carbonate, have been found to lead to toxic effects in adult humans. In untreated cases, doses of 3-5 g (40-70 mg/kg body weight) were lethal.

10.1.2 Toxic effects; dose-effect and dose-response relationships

The absorption of barium from the gastrointestinal tract is largely dependent on age and the solubility of the compound. Less than 10% of the ingested barium is believed to be absorbed in adults. However, absorption may be significantly higher in children. Absorbed barium enters the bloodstream and various soft tissues and is deposited in the bone. The metabolism of barium is similar to that of calcium; unlike calcium, however, barium has no known biological function. Barium can replace calcium in many physiological processes, and it affects nerve and muscle activity.

Barium may cause mild skin and severe eye irritation upon contact. Adverse health effects have been observed in sensitive individuals (e.g., diuresis patients) following exposure to barium as a medical X-ray preparation medium. Several cases of barium poisoning have been reported. Symptoms include acute gastroenteritis, loss of deep reflexes with onset of muscular paralysis, and progressive muscular paralysis.

There is no conclusive evidence that barium compounds, with the exception of barium chromate, are carcinogenic in humans, nor is there any conclusive evidence that barium produces reproductive, embryotoxic, or teratogenic effects in humans.

Early limited epidemiological studies relating exposure to low levels of barium to cardiovascular disease and mortality were inconsistent and inconclusive. In a later epidemiological study, no conclusive evidence of barium-induced effects on blood pressure were revealed. No effects on blood pressure were identified in a short-term study in which volunteers consumed increasing levels of barium up to 10 mg/litre in drinking-water.

Barium inhaled in the workplace has resulted in baritosis. The prevalence of hypertension observed in workers exposed to high levels of airborne barium was significantly higher than in unexposed workers. A dose-related increase in systolic blood pressure was reported in rats exposed to concentrations of barium up to 100 mg/litre.

10.1.3 Risk evaluation

On the basis of the available literature, it can be concluded that, for the general population, barium, at the usual concentrations found in water (especially drinking-water), food, and ambient air, does not constitute any significant health risk. However, for specific subpopulations (elderly or potassium-deficient individuals) and under special circumstances (high water content, occupational exposure etc.) the potential for adverse health effects may exist.

10.2 Evaluation of effects on the environment

Barium is present in the soil at an average concentration of 500 μg/g. Concentrations ranging from 0.04 to 37.0 μg/litre and 7.0 to 15 000 μg/litre have been measured in ocean and fresh waters, respectively. Levels of barium in the air are generally $\leq$ 0.05 μg/m^3.

Soluble barium compounds are capable of being transported through the environment and absorbed by organisms. Barium may accumulate in different parts of the plant.

Barium has been reported to inhibit growth and cellular processes in microorganisms. It has also been observed to affect the development of germinating bacterial spores.

No information on the adverse effects of barium on terrestrial plants or wildlife has been found. No toxic effects due to barium have been reported in aquatic plants at usual concentrations in water. The LC$_{50}$ values for fish in fresh water range from 46 to 78 mg/litre. Barium concentrations of 5.8 mg/litre have been observed to impair reproduction and growth in daphnids.

There is a shortage of data for evaluating the risk to the environment posed by barium. Based on the available information on the toxic effects in daphnids, it appears that barium may represent a risk to populations of some aquatic organisms.

11. RECOMMENDATIONS FOR FURTHER STUDIES

Further research studies on barium in the following areas of environmental and human health effects are recommended:

- bioavailability studies, including solubilization and transport mechanisms;

- hypertension/cardiovascular studies involving the general population and occupationally exposed workers, and related mechanisms of action;

- well-designed epidemiological studies;

- studies on the immunological effects of barium on humans;

- long-term sublethal aquatic toxicity studies;

- monitoring data on environmental exposure to identify areas where protective measures are needed;

- assessment of early indicators of high rate of exposure to barium; biomarker studies (e.g., barium content in hair and urine, serum potassium levels).

12. PREVIOUS EVALUATIONS BY INTERNATIONAL BODIES

The International Agency for Research on Cancer Working Group (IARC, 1980) evaluated the carcinogenicity of barium chromate (VI) and concluded that it is a positive human carcinogen. The carcinogenic property of this compound, however, has been ascribed to the chromium (VI) moiety and not to the barium.

REFERENCES

AHMED, A. & HAMZA, H.M. (1989) Barium sulfate absorption and sensitivity. *Radiology*, 172: 213-214.

AKIYAMA, T. & TOMITA, I. (1973) Preparation and some properties of chromium phosphate ion exchanger. *J. inorg. nucl. Chem.*, 35: 2971-2983.

ALLEN, A.S. (1943) Pa Ping of Kiating paralysis. *Chin. med. J.*, 61: 296-301.

ANDERSON, N.R. & HUME, D.N. (1968) The strontium and barium content of sea water. In: *Trace organics in water*, Washington, DC, American Chemical Society, pp. 296-307 (Advances in Chemistry Series No. 73).

AOAC (1984) *Official methods of analysis of the Association of Official Analytical Chemists*, 14th ed., Arlington, Virginia, Association of Official Analytical Chemists.

ASBELL, M.A. & EAGON, R.G. (1966) The role of multivalent cations in the organization and structure of bacterial cell walls. *Biochem. biophys. Res. Commun.* 22(6): 664-671.

AWWA (1985) An AWWA survey of inorganic contaminants in water supplies. Research and Technology Committee Report. *J. Am. Water Works Assoc.*, May: 67-72.

BACON, M.P. & EDMOND, J.P. (1972) Barium at Geosecs III in the Southwest Pacific. *Earth planet. Sci. Lett.*, 16: 66-74.

BARNES, C.D. & ELTHERINGTON, L.G. (1973) *Drug dosages in laboratory animals - A handbook*, Berkeley, California, University of California Press, p. 53.

BARNETT, P.R., SKOUGSTAD, M.W., & MILLER, K.J. (1969) Chemical characterization of a public water supply. *J. Am. Water Works Assoc.*, 2: 60-67.

BARTLET, J.G., ONDERDONK, A.B., LOUIE, T., KASPER, D.L., & GORBACH, S.L. (1978) A review: Lessons from an animal model of intra-abdominal sepsis. *Arch. Surg.*, 113: 853-857.

BAUER, G.C.H., CARLSSON, A., & LINDQUIST, B. (1956) A comparative study on the metabolism of ^{140}Ba and ^{45}Ca in rats. *Biochem. J.*, 63: 536-542.

BECKER, D.A. (1976) Environmental sample banking - research and methodology. *Trace Subst. environ. Health*, 10: 353-359.

BERNAT, M., CHURCH, T., & ALLEGRE, C.J. (1972) Barium and strontium concentrations in Pacific and Mediterranean sea water profiles by direct isotope dilution mass spectrometry. *Earth planet. Sci. Lett.*, 16: 75-80.

BIESINGER, K.E. & CHRISTENSEN, G.M. (1972) Effects of various metals on survival, growth, reproduction, and metabolism of *Daphnia magna*. *J. Fish Res. Board Can.*, 29: 1691-1700.

BLIGH, P.H. & TAYLOR, D.M. (1963) Comparative studies of the metabolism of strontium and barium in the rat. *Biochem. J.,* **87**: 612-618.

BOLTER, E., TUREKIAN, K.K., & SCHULTZ, D.F. (1964) The distribution of rubidium, cesium and barium in the oceans. *Geochim. Cosmochim. Acta,* **28**: 1459-1466.

BORZELLECA, J.F., CONDIE, L.W., & EGLE, J.L. (1988) Short-term toxicity (one- and ten-day gavage) of barium chloride in male and female rats. *J. Am. Coll. Toxicol.,* **1**(5): 675-685.

BOUTET, C. & CHAISEMARTIN, C. (1973) Propriétés toxiques spécifiques des sels métalliques chez *Austropotamobius pallipes pallipes* et *Orconetes limosus*. *C.R. Soc. Biol. Paris,* **167**: 1933-1938.

BOWEN, H.J.M. (1956) Barium in sea water and marine organisms. *J. Mar. Biol. Assoc. (U.K.),* **35**: 451-460.

BOWEN, H.J.M. (1966) *Trace elements in biochemistry,* New York, Academic Press, p. 19.

BOWEN, H.J.M. & DYMOND, J.A. (1955) Strontium and barium in plants and soils. *Proc. R. Soc. Lond.,* **B144**: 355-368.

BRADFIELD, R. (1932) The concentration of cations in clay soils. *J. Phys. Chem.,* **36**: 340-347.

BRADFORD, G.R. (1971) Trace elements in the water resources of California. *Hilgardia,* **41**(3): 45-53.

BREHM, P., DUNLAP, K., & ECKERT, R. (1978) Calcium-dependent repolarization of paramecium. *J. Physiol.,* **274**: 639-654.

BRENDER, D., STRONG, C.G., & SHEPHERD, J.T. (1970) Effects of acetylstrophanthidin on isolated veins of dogs. *Circ. Res.,* **26**: 547-555.

BRENNIMAN, G.R., NAMEKATA, T., KOJOLA, W.H., CARNOW, B.W., & LEVY, P.S. (1979) Cardiovascular disease death rates in communities with elevated levels of barium in drinking water. *Environ. Res.,* **20**: 318-324.

BRENNIMAN, G.R., KOJOLA, W.H., LEVY, P.S., CARNOW, B.W., & NAMEKATA, T. (1981) High barium levels in public drinking water and its association with elevated blood pressure. *Arch. environ. Health,* **36**: 28-32.

BROOKS, R.R. (1978) Pollution through trace elements. In: Bockris, J.O.M., ed. *Environmental chemistry,* New York, Plenum Press, pp. 429-476.

BROOKS, R.R. (1980) Barium accumulation by demids of the genus *Closterium*. *Br. Phycol. J.,* **15**: 261-264.

BROWNING, E. (1969) *Toxicity of industrial metals,* London, Appleton-Century Crofts.

CALABRESE, E.J. (1977) Excessive barium and radium-226 in Illinois drinking water. *J. environ. Health,* **39**(5): 366-369.

CALABRESE, E.J., CANADA, A.T., & SACCO, C. (1985) Trace elements and public health. *Annu. Rev. public Health,* **6**: 131-146.

CANTELMO, F.R., TAGATZ, M.E., & RANGA RAO, K. (1979) Effect of barite on meiofauna in a flow-through experimental system. *Mar. environ. Res.,* **2**: 301-309.

CARTER, G.A. & WAIN, R.L. (1904) Investigations on fungicides. IX. The fungitoxicity, phytotoxicity, and systemic fungicidal activity of some inorganic salts. *Ann. appl. Biol.,* **53**: 291-309.

CARTWRIGHT, K., SPECHT, S.A., GILKESON, R.H., GRIFFIN, R.A., & LARSON, T.E. (1978) *Geologic studies to identify the source of high levels of radium and barium in Illinois ground water supply: A preliminary report*, Springfield, Virginia, US Department of Commerce, Office of Water Research and Technology, pp. 13, 287, 737.

CASTAGNOU, R., PAOLETTI, C., & LARABEAU, S. (1957) Absorption et répartition de baryum administré par voie intraveineuse ou par voie orale du rat. *C.R. Acad. Sci., Paris,* **24**: 2994.

CENTRO DE INFORMACION TOXICOLOGICA (1972) Treatments for poisonings caused by rodenticides. *Antioquia Med.,* **22**: 699-704.

CHAN, L.H., DRUMMOND, D., EDMOND, J.M., & GRANT, B. (1977) On the barium data from the Atlantic GEOSECS expedition. *Deep Sea Res.,* **24**: 613-649.

CHOW, T.J. (1976) Barium in southern California waters: A potential indicator of marine drilling contamination. *Science,* **193**: 57-58.

CHOW, T.J. & GOLDBERG, E.D. (1960) On the marine geochemistry of barium. *Geochim. Cosmochim. Acta,* **20**: 192-198.

CHOW, T.J. & PATTERSON, C.C. (1966) Concentration profiles of barium and lead in Atlantic waters off Bermuda. *Earth. planet. Sci. Lett.,* **1**: 397-400.

CHOW, T.J., EARL, J.L., REED, J.H., HANSEN, N., & ORPHAN, V. (1978) Barium content of marine sediments near drilling sites: A potential pollutant indicator. *Mar. Pollut. Bull.,* **9**: 97-99.

CLARK, F.W. & WASHINGTON, H.S. (1924) *The composition of the earth's crust,* Washington, DC, US Department of the Interior (US Geological Survey: Professional Paper No. 127).

CLARY, J.J. & TARDIFF, R.G. (1974) The absorption, distribution and excretion of orally administered $^{133}BaCl_2$ in weanling male rats. *Toxicol. appl. Pharmacol.,* **29**: 139.

CLAVEL, J.P., LORRILLOT, M.L., BUTHIAU, D., GERBET, D., HEITZ, F., & GALLI, A. (1987) Intestinal absorption of barium during radiological studies. *Therapie*, 42(2): 239-243.

CONARD, R.A. & SCOTT, W.A. (1961) Modification of radiation-induced gastrointestinal effects of barium meals. *Radiat. Res.*, 15: 527-531.

CONSIDINE, D.M., ed. (1976) *Van Nostrand's scientific encyclopedia*, 5th ed., New York, Van Nostrand Reinhold Company.

COOPER, W.W., BECK, J.N., CHEN, T.S., & KURODA, P.K. (1970) Radioactive strontium and barium fallout. *Health Phys.*, 19: 625-632.

CRAWFORD, A.C. (1908) Barium, a cause of the loco-weed disease. *US Dept. Agric. Bur. Plant Ind. Bull.*, 129: 87.

CRC (1988) CRC Handbook of chemistry and physics, 68th ed., Boca Raton, Florida, Chemical Rubber Publishing Company (CRC).

CREASON, J.P., HINNERS, T.A., BUMGARNER, J.E., & PINKERTON, C. (1975) Trace elements in hair, as related to exposure in metropolitan New York. *Clin. Chem.*, 21: 606-612.

CREASON, J.P., SVENDSGAARD, D., BUMGARNER, J.E., PINKERTON, C., & HINNERS, T.A. (1976) Maternal-fetal tissue levels of 16 trace elements in 8 selected continental United States communities. *Trace Subst. environ. Health*, 10: 53-62.

CUDDIHY, R.G. & GRIFFITH, W.C. (1972) A biological model describing tissue distribution and whole body retention of barium and lanthanum in beagle dogs after inhalation and gavage. *Health Phys.*, 23: 621-633.

CUDDIHY, R.G. & OZOG, J.A. (1973) Nasal absorption of $CsCl$, $SrCL_2$, $BaCl_2$ and $CeCl_3$ in Syrian hamsters. *Health Phys.*, 25: 219-224.

CUDDIHY, R.G., HALL, R.P., & GRIFFITH, W.C. (1974) Inhalation exposures to barium aerosols: Physical, chemical and mathematical analysis. *Health Phys.*, 26: 405-416.

CUFFE, S.T. & GERSTLE, R.W. (1967) *Emissions from coal-fired power plants*, Washington, DC, US Department of Health, Education and Welfare, Government Printing Office (Publication No. 999-AP-35).

CUTRESS, T.W. (1979) A preliminary study of the microelement composition of the outer layer of dental enamel. *Caries Res.*, 13: 73-79.

DARE, P.R., HEWE, H.P.J., HICKS, R., VAN BEMST, A., ZOBER, A., & FLEISHER, M. (1984) Barium in welding fume. *Ann. occup. Hyg.*, 28(4): 445-448.

DAUGHERTY, F.M., Jr (1951) Effects of some chemicals used in oil well drilling on marine animals. *Sewage ind. Wastes*, 23: 1282-1287.

DAVIS, W.E. (1972) *National inventory of sources and emissions: Barium, boron, copper, selenium and zinc*, Washington, DC, US Environmental Protection Agency, p. 56 (EPA 68-02-0100).

DEJONG, L.E. & ROMAN, W.B. (1971) Tolerance of Azobacter for metallic and nonmetallic ions. *J. Microbiol. Serol.*, 37: 119-124.

DENCKER, L., NILLSON, A., RONNBACK, C., & WALINDER, G. (1976) Uptake and retention of ^{133}Ba and ^{140}Ba-^{140}La in mouse tissues. *Acta radiol.*, 15: 273-287.

DEN DOOREN DE JONG, L.E. (1965) Tolerance of *Chlorella vulgaris* for metallic and non-metallic ions. *Antonie van Leeuwenhoek*, 31: 301-313.

DEVI PRASAD, P.V. (1984) Effect of magnesium, strontium and barium on the calcification of the freshwater green alga *Gloeotaenium*. *Phykos*, 23: 202-206.

DIENGOTT, D., ROZSA, O., LEVY, N., & MUAMMAR, S. (1964) Hypokalemia in barium poisoning. *Lancet*, 2: 343-344.

DOIG, A.T. (1976) Baritosis: A benign pneumoconiosis. *Thorax*, 31: 30-39.

DOMANSKI, T.M., DEPCZYK, D., & LINIECKI, J. (1964) A test of the theory of alkaline earth metabolism by the behaviour of ^{133}Ba in rats. *Phys. Med. Biol.*, 11: 461-470.

DOMANSKI, T.M., LINIECKI, J., & WITKOWSKI, D. (1969) Kinetics of calcium, strontium, barium, and radium in rats. In: Mays, C.W., Jee, W.S.W., & Lloyd, R.D., ed. *Delayed effects of bone seeking radionuclides*, Salt Lake City, Utah, University of Utah Press, pp. 81-103.

DOUGLAS, W.W. & POISNER, A.M. (1962) On the mode of action of acetylcholine in evoking adrenal medullary secretion: Increased uptake of calcium during the secretory response. *J. Physiol.*, 162: 385-392.

DOUGLAS, W.W. & RUBIN, R.P. (1963) The mechanism of catecholamine release from the adrenal medulla and the role of calcium in stimulus-secretion coupling. *J. Physiol.*, 167: 288-310.

DOUGLAS, W.W. & RUBIN, R.P. (1964a) Stimulant action of barium on the adrenal medulla. *Nature (Lond.)*, 203: 305-307.

DOUGLAS, W.W. & RUBIN, R.P. (1964b) The effects of alkaline earths and other divalent cations on adrenal medullary secretion. *J. Physiol.*, 175: 231-241.

DURFOR, C.M. & BECKER, E. (1964) *Public water supplies of the 100 largest cities in the United States, 1962*, Washington, DC, US Department of the Interior, Government Printing Office (US Geological Survey: Water Supply Paper No. 1812).

DURUM, W. (1960) Occurrence of trace elements in water. In: Faber, H. & Bryson, L., ed. *Proceedings of the Conference on Physiological Aspects of Water Quality, Washington, DC, 8-9 September, 1960,* Washington, DC, Public Health Service, Division of Water Supply and Pollution Control, Research and Training Grants Branch.

DYBCZYNSKI, R. (1972) Effect of resin cross-linking on the cation-exchange separation of alkali and alkaline earth metals on sulphonic cation exchangers. *J. Chromatogr.,* 71: 507-522.

EINBRODT, H.J., WOBKER, F., & KLIPPEL, H.G. (1972) [Animal experiments on the deposit and distribution of barium sulfate in the rat organism after inhalation.] *Int. Arch. Arbeitsmed.,* 30: 237-244 (in German).

ELLSASSER, J.C., FARNHAM, J.E., & MARSHAL, J.H. (1969) Comparative kinetics and autoradiography of ^{45}Ca and ^{133}Ba in 10-year-old beagle dogs. *J. Bone joint Surg.,* 51: 1397-1412.

ELORZA, M.V. (1969) Toxicity of metal ions to *Aspergillis nidulans. Microbiol. Esp.,* 22: 131-137.

ELWOOD, P.C., ABERNETHY, M., & NORTON, M. (1974) Mortality in adults and trace elements in water. *Lancet,* 2: 1470-1472.

EPSTEIN, M.S. & ZANDER, A.T. (1979) Direct determination of barium in sea and estuarine water by graphite furnace atomic spectrometry. *Anal. Chem.,* 51: 915-918.

ERDELYI, L. (1977) Synaptic activation of Helix ganglion cells by barium ions. *Molecologia,* 16: 93-100.

EVANS, R.B., SNELLING, R.N., & BUCK, F.N. (1973) Assessment of doses in the western United States from the People's Republic of China nuclear test of January 7, 1972. *Radiat. Data Rep.,* 2: 77-83.

FAILYER, G.H. (1910) Barium in soils. *US Dept. Agric. Bur. Soils Bull.,* 72: 23.

FASSEL, V.A. & KNISELEY, R.N. (1974) Inductively coupled plasma optical emission spectrometry. *Anal. Chem.,* 46: 1110A-1120A.

FECZKO, P.J., SIMMS, S.M., BAKIRCI, N. (1989) Fatal hypersensitivity reaction during a barium enema. *Am. J. Radiol.,* 153: 275-276.

FOERSTER, H.F. & FOSTER, J.W. (1966) Endotrophic calcium, strontium, and barium spores of *Bacillus megaterium* and *Bacillus cereus. J. Bacteriol.,* 91: 1333-1335.

FORSSEN, A. & ERAMETSA, O. (1974) Inorganic elements in the human body. Ba, Br, Ca, Cd, K, Ni, Pb, Sn, Sr, Ti, Y and Zn in hair. *Ann. Acad. Sci. Fenn. A.V. Med.,* 162: 1-5.

FORTESCUE, J.A.C., CURTIS, S.A., RICHARDSON, J., & CAMPBELL, J. (1976) Regional geochemical maps for the east end of the Niagara Pennisula. *Trace Subst. environ. Health,* 10: 177-184.

FOSTER, P.R., ELHARRAR, V., & ZIPES, D.P. (1977) Accelerated ventricular escapes induced in the intact dog by barium, strontium and calcium. *J. Pharmacol. exp. Ther.,* 200: 373-383.

FRENCH, N.R. (1963) *Review and discussion of barium in radioecology,* New York, Reinhold Press.

GARBARINO, J.R. & TAYLOR, H.E. (1979) An inductive-coupled plasma atomic-emission spectrometric method for routine water quality testing. *Appl. Spectrosc.,* 33: 220-226.

GARNER, R.J., JONES, H.G., & SAUSOM, B.F. (1960) Fission products and the dairy cow. Some aspects of the metabolism of the alkaline earth elements calcium, strontium, and barium. *Biochem. J.,* 76: 572-579.

GEORGE, R.Y. (1975) Potential effects of oil drilling and dumping activities in marine biota. In: *Proceedings of the Conference on Environmental Aspects of Chemical Use in Well-Drilling Operations, Houston, Texas, May 1975,* Washington, DC, US Environmental Protection Agency, Office of Toxic Substances, pp. 333-335 (EPA 560/1-75-004).

GOLDBERG, E.D.D & ARRHENIUS, G. (1958) Chemistry of Pacific pelagic sediments. *Geochim. Cosmochim. Acta,* 13: 153-212.

GOODENOUGH, R.D. & STENGER, V.A. (1973) Magnesium, calcium, strontium, barium and radium. In: Bailer, J.D., Jr, Emeleus, H.J., & Trotman-Dickinson, J., ed. *Comprehensive inorganic chemistry,* Oxford, Pergamon Press, pp. 591-664.

GOODMAN, L.S. & GILMAN, A. (1980) *The pharmacological basis of therapeutics,* 6th ed., New York, The MacMillan Company.

GORMICAN, A. (1970) Inorganic elements in foods used in hospital menus. *J. Am. Diet. Assoc.,* 56: 397-403.

GOULD, D.B., SORRELL, M.R., & LUPARIELLO, A.D. (1973) Barium sulfide poisoning. Some factors contributing to survival. *Arch. int. Med.,* 132: 891-894.

GRAHAM, C.F. (1934) Barium chloride poisoning. *J. Am. Med. Assoc.,* 102: 1471.

GRANTHAM, C.K. & SLOAN, J.P. (1975) Toxicity study. Drilling fluid chemicals on aquatic life. In: *Proceedings of the Conference on Environmental Aspects of Chemical Use in Well-Drilling Operations, Houston, Texas May 1975,* Washington, DC, US Environmental Protection Agency, Office of Toxic Substances, pp. 103-110 (EPA 560/1-75-004).

GRAY, C., SIVALOGANATHAN, S., & SIMPKINS, K.C. (1989) Aspiration of high-density barium contrast medium causing acute pulmonary inflammation - Report of two fatal cases in elderly women with disordered swallowing. *Clin. Radiol.,* **40**: 397-400.

GREBECKI, A. & KUZNICKI, L. (1963) The influence of external pH on the toxicity of inorganic ions for *P. candatum. Acta Protozool.,* **1**: 157-184.

GUDIKSEN, P.H., CHAKRAVARTI, D., FAIRHALL, A.W., & YOUNG, J.A. (1965) Debris from the Chinese atomic test of May 1965, intercepted over the northwestern United States. *Health Phys.,* **12**: 862-863.

GUPTA, S.R., PRASANNA, H.R., VISWANATHAN, W., & VENKITASUBRAMANIAN, T.A. (1975) Effect of inorganic salts and some biologically important compounds on the incorporation of acetate-1-^{14}C into aflatoxins by resting mycelia of *Aspergillis parasiticus. Z. Lebensm. Unters. Forsch.,* **157**: 19-22.

GUTHRIE, R.K., DAVIS, E.M., CHERRY, S., & MURRAY, H.E. (1979) Biomagnification of heavy metals by organisms in a marine microcosm. *J. environ. Contam. Toxicol.,* **21**: 53-61.

GUTWEIN, E.E., LANDOLT, R.R., & BRENCHLEY, D.L. (1974) Barium retention in rats exposed to combustion products from diesel fuel containing a barium-based antismoke additive. *J. Air. Pollut. Control Assoc.,* **24**(1): 40-43.

HAMILTON, E.I. & MINSKI, M.J. (1972) Abundance of the chemical element in man's diet and possible relations with environmental factors. *Sci. Environ.,* **1**: 315.

HANSEN, M. (1958) *Constitution of binary alloys,* New York, McGraw-Hill Book Company, Inc.

HARRISON, G.E., CARR, T.E.F., SUTTON, A., & RUNDO, J. (1966) Plasma concentration and excretion of calcium-47, strontium-85, barium-133 and radium-223 following successive intravenous doses to a healthy man. *Nature (Lond.),* **209**: 526-527.

HARRISON, G.E., CARR, T.E.F. & SUTTON, A. (1967) Distribution of radioactive calcium, strontium, barium and radium following intravenous injection into a healthy man. *Int. J. Radiat. Biol.,* **13**: 235-247.

HAUSLER, G. & HAEFELY, W. (1979) Modification of release by adrenergic neutron blocking agents and agents that alter the action potential. In: Paton, D.M., ed. *The release of catecholamines from adrenergic neutrons,* New York, Pergamon Press, pp. 185-216.

HAVLIK, B., HANUSOVA, J., & RALKOVA, J. (1980) Hygienic importance of increased barium content in some fresh waters. *J. Hyg. Epidemiol. Microbiol. Immunol.,* **24**(4): 396-404.

HAWLEY, G.G. (1977) *The condensed chemical dictionary,* 9th ed., New York, Van Nostrand Reinhold Company.

HEFFRON, C.L., REID, J.T., & FURR, A.K. (1977) Lead and other elements in sheep fed colored magazines and newsprint. *J. agric. food Chem.*, 25: 657-660.

HEITMULLER, P.T., HOLLISTER, T.A., & PARRISH, P.R. (1981) Acute toxicity of 54 industrial chemicals to sheepshead minnows *(Cyprinodon variegatus)*. *Bull. environ. Contam. Toxicol.*, 27: 596-604.

HELDMAN, E., LEVINE, M., RAVEH, L., & POLLARD, H.B. (1989) Barium ions enter chromaffin cells via voltage-dependent calcium channels and induce secretion by a mechanism independent of calcium, *J. biol. Chem.*, 264(14): 7914-7920.

HENDERSON, E.G. & VOLLE, R.L. (1972) Ion exchange in frog sartorious muscle treated with 9-aminoacridine or barium. *J. Pharmacol. exp. Ther.*, 183: 356-369.

HICKS, R., CALDAS, L.Q., DARE, P.R., & HEWITT, P.J. (1986) Cardiotoxic and bronchoconstrictor effects of industrial metal fumes containing barium. *Arch. Toxicol.*, Suppl. 9: 416-420.

HILDEBRAND, S.G., CUSHMAN, R.M., & CARTER, J.A. (1976) The potential toxicity and bioaccumulation in aquatic systems of trace elements present in aqueous coal conversion effluents. In: Hemphill, D.D., X, ed., *Trace substances in environmental health,* Columbia, Missouri, University of Missouri.

HIRANO, Y. & HIRAOKA, M. (1986) Changes in K^+ current induced by Ba^{2+} in guinea pig ventricular muscles. *Am. J. Physiol.*, 251: 24-33.

IARC (1973) *Some inorganic and organometallic compounds,* Lyon, International Agency for Research on Cancer, p. 102 (IARC Monographs on the Evaluation of Carcinogenic Risk of Chemicals to Humans, Vol. 2).

IARC (1980) *Some metals and metallic compounds,* Lyon, International Agency for Research on Cancer, p. 205 (IARC Monographs on the Evaluation of the Carcinogenic Risk of Chemicals to Humans, Vol. 23).

IARC (1987) Chromium and chromium compounds: Chromium metal, trivalent chromium compounds, hexavalent chromium compounds. In: Overall evaluations of carcinogenicity: An updating of IARC Monographs Volumes 1 to 42, Lyon, International Agency for Research on Cancer, pp. 165-168 (IARC Monographs on the Evaluation of Carcinogenic Risks to Humans, Supplement 7).

ICRP (INTERNATIONAL COMMISSION ON RADIOLOGICAL PROTECTION) (1959) *Recommendations of the International Commission on Radiological Protection. Report of Committee II,* Elmsford, New York, Pergamon Press (ICRP Publication No. 2).

ICRP (1974) *Report of the Task Group on Reference Man. A report prepared by a task group of Committee 2 of the International Commission on Radiological Protection,* Oxford, New York, Pergamon Press (ICRP Report No. 23).

ICRP (INTERNATIONAL COMMISSION ON RADIOLOGICAL PROTECTION) (1975) Report of the Task Group on Reference Man, No. 23. Pergamon Press, Elmsford, New York.

IZMEROV, N.F., SANOTSKY, I.V., & SIDEROV, K.K. (1982) *Toxicometric parameters of industrial toxic chemicals under single exposure*, Moscow, Centre of International Projects, GKNT, p. 23.

IZUMI, F., TOYOHIRA, Y., YANAGIHARA, N., WADA, A., & KOBAYASHI, H. (1986) Barium evoked release of cuthecholamines from digitonin-premeabilized adrenal medullary cells. *Neuro-Sci. Lett.*, **69**: 172-175.

KASSANIS, B., WHITE, R.F., & WOODS, R.D. (1975) Inhibition of multiplication of tobacco mosaic virus in protoplasts by antibiotics and its prevention by divalent metals. *J. gen. Virol.*, **28**: 185-191.

KATZUNG, B.G. & MORGENSTERN, J. (1976) The effects of potassium and barium on ventricular automaticity and the pacemaker current. *Proc. West. Pharmacol. Soc.*, **19**: 299-302.

KELLEY, K.K. (1933) *Contribution to the data on theoretical metallurgy. II. High-temperature specific-heat equation for inorganic substances*, Pittsburg, Pennsylvania, US Bureau of Mines (Bulletin No. 371).

KINOSITA, H., DRYL, S., & NAITOH, Y. (1964) Spontaneous change in membrane potential of *Paramecium caudatum* induced by barium and calcium ions. *Bull. Acad. Pol. Sci. Ser. Sci. Biol.*, **12**: 459-461.

KIRPEKAR, S.M. & MISU, Y. (1967) Release of noradrenaline by splenic nerve stimulation and its dependence on calcium. *J. Physiol.*, **188**: 219-234.

KIRPEKAR, S.M., PRAT, J.C., PUIG, M., & WAKADE, A.R. (1972) Modification of the evoked release of noradrenaline from the perfused cat spleen by various ions and agents. *J. Physiol.*, **221**: 601-615.

KNOP, W. (1874) Analyses of the Nile sediment. *Landwirtsch. Vers.-Stn*, **17**: 65-70.

KOIRTYOHANN, S.R. & PICKETT, E.E. (1968) The nitrous oxide-acetylene flame in emission analysis - II. Lithium and the alkaline earths. *Spectroclin. Acta*, **23B**: 673-685.

KOJOLA, W.H., BRENNIMAN, G.R., & CARNOW, B.W. (1978) A review of environmental characteristics and health effects of barium in public water supplies. *Rev. environ, Health*, **3**(1): 79-95.

KOLPAKOV, V.V. (1971) Effect of barium chloride on production of humoral factors stimulating leukopoiesis. *Patol. Fiziol. eksp. Ter.*, **5**(6): 64-66.

KONONENKO, K.I. & CHAIKINA, L.A. (1970) Effect of metal ion in the electric charge of cells. *Biofizika*, **15**: 1127-1129.

KOPP, J. (1969) The occurrence of trace elements in water. In: Hemphill, D.D., III, ed. *Trace substances in environmental health*, Columbia, Missouri, University of Missouri, pp. 59-73.

KOPP, J.F. & KRONER, R.C. (1967) Tracing water pollution with an emission spectrograph. *J. Water Pollut. Control Fed.*, **39**: 1659.

KOPP, J.F. & KRONER, R.C. (1968) A comparison of trace elements in natural waters, dissolved vs. suspended. *Dev. appl. Spectrosc.*, **6**: 339-352.

KOPP, J.F. & KRONER, R.C. (1970) *Trace metals in waters of the United States: A five-year summary of trace metals in rivers and lakes of the United States (1 October 1962 - 30 September 1967)*, Cincinnati, Ohio, US Department of the Interior, Federal Water Pollution Control Administration, Division of Pollution Surveillance.

KOPP, S.J., PERRY, H.M., Jr., FELIKSIK, J., ERLANGER, M., & PERRY, E. (1985) Cardiovascular dysfunction and hypersensitivity to sodium pentobarbital induced by chronic barium chloride ingestion. *Toxicol. appl. Pharmacol.*, **72**: 303-314.

KOSHI, Y. (1966) Mechanism of cell fusion caused by the haemagglutinating virus of Japan: Requirement of calcium for cell fusion. *Nara Joshi Daigaku Seibutsu Gakkaishi*, **16**: 25-28.

KOVALSKII, V.V., BOROVIK, T.F., LETUNOVA, S.V., & GINZBURG, E.O. (1965) Level of trace elements in microorganisms. *Mikrobiologiya*, **34**: 403-406.

LANGE, N.A. (1985) *Lange's handbook of chemistry*, 10th ed., New York, McGraw Hill Publishers, pp. 425-427.

LEBEDENA, ZH.D., VOLKOVA, I.M., & RUBAN, E.L. (1976) Effect of metal ions on the lipolytic activity of *M. rubrum* and *A. streptomycini*. *Mikrobiologiya*, **45**: 104-110.

LEBLANC, G.A. (1980) Acute toxicity of priority pollutants to water flea (*Daphnia magna*). *Bull. environ. Contam. Toxicol.*, **24**: 684-691.

LEDEBO, I. (1976) Divalent cations in the envelope of a psychrophilic Archromobacter. *J. gen. Microbiol.*, **94**: 351-358.

LEDERER, C.M., HOLLANDER, J.M., & PERLMAN, I. (1967) *Table of the isotopes*, 6th ed., New York, John Wiley and Sons.

LEE, E.G.H., TOWNSLEY, P.M., & WALDEN, C.C. (1966) Effects of bivalent cations on the production of aflatoxins in submerged cultures. *J. food Sci.*, **31**: 432-436.

LESLIE, S.W. & BOROWITZ, J.L. (1975) Inhibition of the adrenal chromaffin and membrane calcium by caffeine and various divalent anions. *Res. Commun. chem. Pathol. Pharmacol.*, **11**: 413-424.

LETKIEWICZ, F., SPOONER, C., MACULUSO, C., & BROWN, D. (1984) *Occurrence of barium in drinking water, food and oil*, Washington, DC, US Environmental Protection Agency, Office of Drinking Water.

LEWI, Z. & BAR-KHAYIM, Y. (1964) Food poisoning from barium carbonate. *Lancet*, 2: 342-343.

LILOV, L. & ZAHN, D. (1967) Effects of some cations on the hydrogenase activity of *Proteus vulgaris* OX 19. *Zentralbl. Bakteriol.*, 121: 475-478.

LINIECKI, J. & KARNEWICZ, W. (1971) Long term retention of radiobarium and radiostrontium in rabbits. *Nukleonika (Warsaw)*, 16: 591-604.

LOSEE, F.L., CUTRESS, T.W., & BROWN, R. (1974) Natural elements of the periodic table in human dental enamel. *Caries Res.* 8: 123-134.

MCCABE, L. (1974) Problems of trace metals in water supplies - an overview. In: Saponzik, A., ed. *Proceedings of the 16th Water Quality Conference on Trace Metals in Water Supplies: Occurrence, Significance and Control, Urbana, Illinois, University of Illinois, 12-13 February 1974*, pp. 1-9.

MCCABE, L.J., SYMONS, J.M., LEE, R.D., & ROBECK, G.C. (1970) Survey of community water supply systems. *J. Am. Water Works Assoc.*, 62: 670-687.

MCCAULEY, P.T. & WASHINGTON, I.S. (1983) Barium bioavailability as the chloride, sulfate, or carbonate salt in the rat. *Drug chem. Toxicol.*, 6: 209-217.

MCCAULEY, P.T., DOUGLAS, B.H., LAURIE, R.D., & BULL, R.J. (1985) Investigations into the effect of drinking water barium on rats. In: *Advances in modern environmental toxicology*, Princeton, New Jersey, Princeton Publishing Co., Vol. IX, pp. 197-210.

MCHARGUE, J.S. (1913) The occurrence of barium in tobacco and other plants. *Am. Chem. Soc. J.*, 35: 826-834.

MCLACHLAN, E.M. (1977) The effects of strontium and barium ions at synapses in sympathetic ganglia. *J. Physiol.*, 267: 497-518.

MCMICHAEL, J.C. & LAUFFER, M.A. (1975) A specific effect of calcium ion on the polymerization-depolymerization of tobacco mosaic virus protein. *Arch. Biochem. Biophys.*, 169: 209-216.

MAGILL, W.A. & SVEHLA, G. (1974) Study on the elimination of interferences in the determination of barium by atomic absorption spectrophotometry. *Z. anal. Chem.*, 268: 180-184.

MARSH, D.D., ALSBERG, C.L., & BLACK, O.F. (1912) The relation of barium to the loco-weed disease. *US Dept. Agric. Plant Indus. Bull.*, 246: 67.

MARUTA, T., TAKEUCHI, T., & SUZUKI, M. (1972) Spectrophotometric studies on 5,7-dibromo-8-aminoquinoline chelates of some bivalent transition metals. *Anal. chem. Acta*, 58: 452-455.

MEIER, C.F., Jr & KATZUNG, B.G. (1978) Effects of cesium and barium on depolarization: Induced automaticity in ventricular myocardium. *Proc. West. Pharmacol. Soc.*, 21: 71-75.

MILLER, R.G., FEATHERSTONE, J.D.B., CARZON, M.E.J., MILLS, T.S., & SHIELDS, C.P. (1985) Barium in teeth as indicator of body burden. In: Advances in modern environmental toxicology, Princeton, New Jersey, Princeton Publishing Company, Vol. 9, pp. 211-219.

MINER, S. (1969) *Air pollution aspects of barium and its compounds*, Bethesda, Maryland, Litton Systems, Inc., Environmental System Division, p. 63. (NTIS PB-188083).

MORROW, P.E., GIBB, F.R., & JOHNSON, L. (1964) Clearance of insoluble dust from the lower respiratory tract. *Health Phys.*, 10: 543-555.

MORTON, M.S., ELWOOD, P.C., & AVERNETHY, M. (1976) Trace elements in water and congenital malformations of the central nervous system in South Wales. *Br. J. Soc. Med.*, 30: 36-39.

MORTON, W. (1945) Poisoning by barium carbonate. *Lancet*, 2: 738-739.

MURPHY, E.W., PAGE, L., & WATT, B.K. (1971) Trace minerals in type A school lunches. *J. Am. Diet. Assoc.*, 59: 115-122.

NADKARNI, R.A. & MORRISON, G.H. (1974) Multi-element analysis of sludge samples by instrumental neutron activation analysis. *Environ. Lett.*, 6: 273-285.

NAS (1977) *Drinking water and health*, Washington, DC, National Academy of Sciences, Printing and Publication Office.

NIOSH (1976) *Health hazard evaluation and determination report. B.F. Goodrich Company, Koroseal Division, Marietta, Ohio*, Cincinnati, Ohio, National Institute for Occupational Safety and Health, Center for Disease Control (NIOSH Report No. 75-24-273).

NIOSH (1977) *NIOSH manual of analytical methods. Standards program validated methods. III.*, Cincinnati, Ohio, National Institute for Occupational Safety and Health, p. 5198.

NIOSH (1978) *Health hazard evaluation determination report: Mark Steel Corporation, Salt Lake City, Utah*, Cincinnati, Ohio, National Institute for Occupational Safety and Health, Center for Disease Control (NIOSH Report No. 78-93-536).

NIOSH (1979) *Health hazard evaluation and technical assistance report: Kentile Floors Inc., South Plainfield, New Jersey*, Cincinnati, Ohio, National Institute for Occupational Safety and Health, Center for Disease Control (NIOSH Report No. 78-72-618).

NIOSH (1980) *Technical assistance report*, Cincinnati, Ohio, National Institute for Occupational Safety and Health, Center for Disease Control (NIOSH Report No. 79-022-789).

References

NIOSH (1982) *Health hazard evaluation report: Sherwin Williams Company, Coffeyille, Kansas,* Cincinnati, Ohio, National Institute for Occupational Safety and Health, Center for Disease Control (NIOSH Report No. HETA/81-356-1183).

NIOSH (1984) *Industrial hygiene survey report of Dorchester Refining Company, 15 September - 5 October, 1981,* Cincinnati, Ohio, National Institute for Occupational Safety and Health, Center for Disease Control (NIOSH Report No. 124-11).

NIOSH (1985) *Health hazard evaluation report: General Motors Corporation, Dayton, Ohio,* Cincinnati, Ohio, National Institute for Occupational Safety and Health, Center for Disease Control (NIOSH Report No. HETA/84-060-1645).

NIOSH (1987a) *NIOSH manual of analytical methods. Standards completion program validated methods. Barium methods 7056,* Cincinnati, Ohio, National Institute for Occupational Safety and Health, Center for Disease Control.

NIOSH (1987b) *Health hazard evaluation report: Wellman Dynamics Corporation, Creston, Iowa,* Cincinnati, Ohio, National Institute for Occupational Safety and Health, Center for Disease Control (NIOSH Report No. HETA/83-015-1809).

NIOSH (1987c) *Health hazard evaluation report: International Association of Fire Fighters, Washington, DC,* Cincinnati, Ohio, National Institute for Occupational Safety and Health, Center for Disease Control (NIOSH Report No. HETA/85-540-1816).

NISHIOKA, H. (1975) Mutagenic activities of metal compounds in bacteria. *Mutat. Res.,* **31**: 186-189.

PAPPANO, A.J. (1976) Action potentials in chick atria: Ontogenetic changes in the dependence of tetrodotoxin-resistent action potentials on calcium, strontium and barium. *Circ. Res.,* **39**(1): 99-105.

PARANCHYCH, W. (1966) Stages in phage R17 infection. *Virology,* **28**: 90-99.

PCOC (1966) *Pesticide chemical official compendium,* Topeka, Kansas, Association of the American Pesticide Control Officials, Inc., p. 95.

PENDERGRASS, E.P. & GREENING, R.R. (1953) Baritosis: report of a case. *Arch. ind. Hyg. occup. Med.,* **7**: 44-48.

PENTO, J.T. (1979) The influence of barium on calcitonin secretion in the pig. *Pharmacol. Res. Commun.,* **11**: 221-226.

PERRY, H.M., Jr & YUNICE, A. (1965) Acute pressure effects of intraarterial cadmium and mercuric ions in anesthetized rats. *Proc. Soc. Exp. Biol. Med.,* **120**: 805-808.

PERRY, H.M., Jr., TIPTON, I.H., SCHROEDER, H.A., & COOK, M.J. (1962) Variability in the metal content of human organs. *J. lab. clin. Med.,* **60**: 245-253.

PERRY, H.M., SCHOEPFLE, E., & BOURGOIGNIE, J. (1967) *In vitro* production and inhibition of aortic vasoconstriction by mercuric, cadmium, and other metal ions. *Proc. Soc. Exp. Biol. Med.*, **124**: 485-490.

PERRY, H.M., KOPP, S.Y., ERLANGER, M.W., & PERRY, E.F. (1983) Cardiovascular effects of chronic barium ingestion. In: Hemphill, D.D., ed. *Trace substances in environmental health*, Columbia, Missouri, University of Missouri, pp. 155-164.

PERRY, H.M., PERRY, E.F., ERLANGER, M.W., & KOPP, S.J. (1985) Barium induced hypertension. In: Calabrese, E., ed. *Inorganics in drinking water and cardiovascular disease*, Princeton, New Jersey, Princeton Publishing Co., Chapter 20, pp. 221-229.

PETERSON, D.T. & INDIG, M. (1960) The barium-barium hydride phase system. *J. Am. Chem. Soc.*, **82**: 5645-5646.

PEYTON, J.C. & BOROWITZ, J.L. (1978) Effects of Ba^{2+} and Cd^{2+} on convulsive electroshock sensitivity and ^{45}Ca distribution in brain subcellular fractions in mice. *Toxicol. appl. Pharmacol.*, **45**: 95-103.

PHELAN, D.M., HAGLEY, S.R., & GUERIN, M.D. (1984) Is hypokalaemia the cause of paralysis in barium poisoning? *Br. med. J.*, **289**: 882.

PIERCE, F.D. & BROWN, H.R. (1977) A semi-automated technique for the separation and determination of barium and strontium in surface waters by ion exchange chromatography and atomic emission spectrometry. *Anal. Lett.*, **10**: 685-699.

PIERSON, W.R., TRUEX, T.J., MCKEE, D.E., SHELEF, M., & BAKER, R.E. (1981) Effects of barium fuel additive and fuel sulfur level on diesel exhaust. *Environ. Sci. Technol.*, **14**(9): 1121-1124.

POPOVA, O.Y.A. & PERETOLCYINA, N.M. (1976) Embryotropic effect of barium fluoride. *Gig. i Sanit.*, **41**: 109-111.

PRONIN, D.A. & PASHKOVSKII, V.G. (1973) Change of the electrical activity of the heart of workers exposed to barium salts. *Gig. Tr. prof. Zabol.*, **17**: 36-37.

QUAGLIANO, J.V. (1959) *Chemistry*, Englewood, New Jersey, Prentice Hall, Inc.

RAE, T. (1977) Tolerance of mouse macrophages *in vitro* to barium sulfate used in orthopedic bone cement. *J. biomed. Mater. Res.*, **11**: 839-846.

RASTORFER, J.R. (1974) Element contents of three Alaskan-Arctic mosses. *Ohio J. Sci.*, **74**: 55-59.

REEVES, A.L. (1979) Barium (toxicity). In: Friberg, L., Nordberg, G.F., & Velimir, B., ed. *Handbook on the toxicology of metals*, Amsterdam, Oxford, New York, Elsevier Science Publishers, pp. 321-328.

REEVES, A.L. (1986) Barium. In: Friberg, L., Nordberg, G.F., & Velimir, B., ed. *Handbook on the toxicology of metals - Volume II: Specific metals*, Amsterdam, Oxford, New York, Elsevier Science Publishers, pp. 84-93.

REISNER, A.H., BUCHOLTZ, C., & CHANDLER, B.S. (1975) Studies on the polyribosomes of paramecium. *Exp. cell Res.*, 93: 1-14.

REZINK, R.B. & TOY, P.A. (1978) *Source assessment: Major barium compounds*, Dayton, Ohio, Monsanto Research Corporation (NTIS PB-280756).

RIDGEWAY, L.P. & KARNOFSKY, D.A. (1952) The effects of metals on the chick embryo: Toxicity and production of abnormalities in development. *Ann. NY Acad. Sci.*, 55: 203-215.

ROBINSON, W.O., WHETSTONE, R.R., & EDGINGTON, G. (1950) The occurrence of barium in soils and plants. *US Dept. Agric. tech. Bull*, 1013: 1-36.

RODE, L.J. & FOSTER, J.W. (1966) Influence of exchangeable ions on germinability of bacterial spores. *J. Bacteriol.*, 91: 1582-1588.

ROUF, M.A. (1964) Spectrochemical analysis of inorganic elements in bacteria. *J. Bacteriol.*, 88: 1545-1549.

ROZA, O. & BERMAN, L.B. (1971) The pathophysiology of barium: Hypokalemic and cardiovascular effects. *J. Pharmacol. exp. Ther.*, 177: 433-439.

RTECS (1985) *Registry of toxic effects of chemical substances. 1983-1984 Cumulative supplement to the 1981-82 edition*. Cincinnati, Ohio, National Institute for Occupational Safety and Health (NIOSH Publication No. 86-103).

RUBIN, R.P. (1970) The role of calcium in the release of neurotransmitter substances and hormones. *Pharmacol. Rev.*, 22: 389-428.

SCHOFIELD, J.G. & COLE, E.N. (1971) Behaviour of systems releasing growth hormones *in vitro*. In: Memoirs of the Society for Endocrinology, pp. 185-201.

SCHROEDER, H.A. (1970) *Barium*, Washington, DC, American Petroleum Institute (Air Quality Monograph No. 70-12).

SCHROEDER, H.A. & KRAEMER, L.A. (1974) Cardiovascular mortality, municipal water and corrosion. *Arch. environ. Health*, 28: 303-311.

SCHROEDER, H.A. & MITCHENER, M. (1975a) Life-term studies in rats: Effects of aluminum, barium, beryllium and tungsten. *J. Nutr.*, 105: 421-427.

SCHROEDER, H.A. & MITCHENER, M. (1975b) Life-term effects of mercury, methyl mercury and nine other trace metals on mice. *J. Nutr.*, 105: 452-458.

SCHROEDER, H.A., TIPTON, I.H., & NASON, A.P. (1972) Trace metals in man: strontium and barium. *J. chron. Dis.*, 25: 491-517.

SEATON, A., RUCKELY, V.A., ADDISON, J., & BROWN, W.R. (1986) Silicons in barium miners. *Thorax*, 41(8): 591-595.

SHANBAKY, I.O., BOROWITZ, J.L., & KESSLER, W.V. (1978) Mechanism of cadmium- and barium-induced adrenal catecholamine release. *Toxicol. appl. Pharmacol.*, **44**: 99-105.

SHANKLE, R. & KEANE, J.R. (1988) Acute paralysis from inhaled barium carbonate. *Arch. Neurol.*, **45**: 579-580.

SHINE, K.I., DOUGLAS, A.M., & RICCHIUTI, N.V. (1978) Calcium, strontium and barium movements during ischemia and reperfusion in rabbit ventricle. *Circ. Res.*, **43**: 712-720.

SHREVE, N.R. (1967) *Chemical process in industries*, 3rd ed., New York, McGraw-Hill, pp. 357-358, 437-444.

SILAYEV, A.A. & TARASENKO, N.Y. (1976) The effect of barium on the generative function and its hygienic significance. *Gig. Tr. prof., Zabol.*, **7**: 33-37.

SILINSKY, E.M. (1978) On the role of barium in supporting the asynchronous release of acetylcholine quanta by motor nerve impulses. *J. Physiol.*, **274**: 157-171.

SILLEN, L.G. & MARTELL, A.E. (1964) *Stability constants of metal-ion complexes*, London, Chemical Society, p. 754 (Special Publication No. 17).

SIROVER, M.A. & LOEB, L.A. (1976a) Metal activation of DNA synthesis. *Biochem. Biophys. Res. Commun.*, **70**: 812-817.

SIROVER, M.A. & LOEB, L.A. (1976b) Infidelity of DNA synthesis *in vitro:* Screening for potential metal mutagens or carcinogens. *Science*, **194**: 1434-1436.

SLATER, C.S., HOLMES, R.S., & BYERS, H.G. (1937) Trace elements in the soils from the erosion experiment stations, with supplementary data on other soils. *US Dept. Agric. tech. Bull.*, **522**: 23.

SLAVICEK, J. (1972) Effect of Ba^{2+} on contractibility of the isolated right rat ventricle. Substitution of NaCl for choline of hypertonic sucrose. *Physiol. Bohemoslov.*, **21**: 189-199.

SLAVIN, W. (1984) *Graphite furnace AAS - A source book*, Norwalk, Connecticut, Perkin-Elmer Corporation.

SMITH, K.A. (1971a) The comparative uptake and translocation by plants of calcium, strontium, barium and radium. I. *Bertholletia excelsa* (Brazil nut tree). *Plant Soil*, **34**: 369-379.

SMITH, K.A. (1971b) The comparative uptake and translocation by plants of calcium, strontium, barium and radium. II. *Triticum vulgare* (wheat). *Plant Soil*, **34**: 643-651.

SMITH, R.P. & GOSSELIN, R.E. (1976) Current concepts about the treatment of selected poisonings. Nitrite, cyanide, sulfide, barium, and quinide. *Annu. Rev. Pharmacol. Toxicol.*, **16**: 189-199.

SOLLMAN, T.A. (1953) *Manual of pharmacology*, Philadelphia, Pennsylvania, W.B. Saunders Co.

SOWDEN, E.M. & PIRIE, A. (1958) Barium and strontium concentrations in eye tissue. *Biochem. J.*, 70: 716-717.

SOWDEN, E.M. & STITCH, S.R. (1957) Trace elements in human tissue. II. Estimation of the concentration of stable strontium and barium in human bone. *Biochem. J.*, 67: 104-109.

SPRITZER, A.A. & WATSON, J.A. (1964) The measurement of ciliary clearance in the lungs of rats. *Health Phys.*, 10: 1093-1097.

STANLEY, R.A. (1974) Toxicity of heavy metals and salts to Eurassian watermilfoil *(Myriophyllum spicatum L.)*. *Arch. environ. Contam. Toxicol.*, 2: 331-341.

STARY, J., KRATZER, K., & PRASILOVA, J. (1984) The accumulation of radium, barium and lead in algae. *J. radioanal. nucl. Chem.*, 84: 17-21.

STOCKHAM, J.D. (1971) The composition of glass furnace emissions. *J. Air Pollut. Control. Assoc.*, 21(11): 713-715.

STOKINGER, H.E. (1981) Chapter 29: The metals. In: *Patty's industrial hygiene and toxicology*, 3rd ed., New York, John Wiley and Sons, Vol. 2A, pp. 1493-2060.

SUBRAMANIAN, K.S. & MERANGER, J.C. (1984) A survey for sodium, potassium, barium, arsenic, and selenium in Canadian drinking water supplies. *At. Spectrosc.*, 5: 34-37.

SYED, I.B. & HOSAIN, F. (1972) Determination of LD_{50} of barium chloride and allied agents. *Toxicol. appl. Pharmacol.*, 25: 150-152.

TABOR, E.C. & WARREN, W.V. (1958) Distribution of certain metals in the atmosphere of some American cities. *Arch. ind. Health*, 17: 145-151.

TANDON, S.P. & MISHRA, M.M. (1968) Activity of nitrifying bacteria in clay-mineral media. Allahabad, India, University of Allahabad, pp. 1-6 (University of Allahabad Studies, Chemistry Section).

TARASENKO, N.Y., PRONIN, O.A., & SILAYEV, A.A. (1977) Barium compounds as industrial poisons (an experimental study). *J. Hyg. Epidemiol. Microbiol. Immunol.*, 21: 361-373.

TARDIFF, R.G., ROBINSON, M., & ULMER, N.S. (1980) Subchronic oral toxicity of $BaCl_2$ in rats. *J. environ. Pathol. Toxicol.*, 4: 267-275.

TAYLOR, D.M., BLIGH, P.H., & DUGGAN, M.H. (1962) The absorption of calcium, strontium, barium and radium from the gastrointestinal tract of the rat. *Biochem. J.*, 83: 25-29.

TAYLOR, N.W. & ORTON, W.L. (1973) Effect of alkaline earth metal salts on flocculence in *S. cerevisiae*. *J. Inst. Brew. (Lond.)*, 79: 294-297.

THOMAS, R.G., EWING, W.C., CATRON, D.L., & MCCLELLAN, R.O. (1973) In vivo solubility of four forms of barium determined by scanning techniques. *Am. Ind. Hyg. Assoc. J.*, **34**: 350-359.

TIPTON, I.H. & COOK, M.J. (1963) Trace elements in human tissue. Part II. Adult subjects from the United States. *Health Phys.*, **9**: 103-145.

TIPTON, I.H., COOK, M.J., STEINER, R.L., BOYE, C.A., PERRY, H.M., Jr, & SCHROEDER, H.A. (1963) Trace elements in human tissue. Part I. Methods. *Health Phys.*, **9**: 89-101.

TIPTON, I.H., SCHROEDER, H.A., PERRY, H.M., Jr, & COOK, M.J. (1965) Trace elements in human tissue. Part III. Subjects from Africa, the Near and Far East and Europe. *Health Phys.*, **11**: 403-451.

TIPTON, I.H., STEWART, P.L., & MARTIN, P.G. (1966) Trace elements in diets and excreta. *Health Phys.*, **12**: 1683-1689.

TIPTON, I.H., STEWART, P.L., & DICKSON, J. (1969) Patterns of elemental excretion in long term balance studies. *Health Phys.*, **16**: 455-462.

TOGATZ, M.E. & TOBIA, M. (1978) Effect of barite ($BaSO_4$) on development of estuarine communities. *Estuarine coastal mar. Sci.* **7**: 401-407.

TOISTER, Z. & LOYTER, A. (1970) Virus-induced fusion of chicken erythrocytes. *Biochem. biophys. Res. Commun.*, **41**: 1523-1530.

TSAI, F., BUCHANAN, E.B., Jr, & DRAKE, L. (1978) The analysis of sediments from the Iowa River. *Sci. total Environ.*, **9**: 277-285.

TUREKIAN, K.K. (1965) Barium in ocean water profiles. *Trans. Am. Geophys. Union,* **46**: 168.

UNDERWOOD, E.J. (1977) *Trace elements in human and animal nutrition,* New York, Academic Press.

US BUREAU OF MINES (1976) *Minerals yearbook,* Washington, DC, US Bureau of Mines.

US EPA (1974) *Methods for chemical analysis of water and wastes,* Cincinnati, Ohio, US Environmental Protection Agency, Environmental Monitoring and Support Laboratory, Environmental Research Center (EPA 625/6-74-003a).

US EPA (1976) *Quality criteria for water,* Washington, DC, US Environmental Protection Agency (EPA 440/9-76-023).

US EPA (1979a) *Methods for chemical analysis of water and wastes,* Cincinnati, Ohio, US Environmental Protection Agency, Environmental Monitoring and Support Laboratory, Office of Research and Development (EPA 600/4-79-020).

US EPA (1979b) *Health consequences of sulfur oxides: A report from CHESS, 1970, 1971,* Research Triangle Park, North Carolina, US Environmental Protection Agency, Environmental Research Center.

References

US EPA (1984) *Health effects assessment for barium.* Cincinnati, Ohio, US Environmental Protection Agency, Office of Health and Environmental Assessment, Environmental Criteria and Assessment Office (Prepared for the Office of Emergency and Remedial Responsible, Washington, DC) (EPA 540/1-86-021).

US EPA (1985) *Integrated risk information system (IRIS). Reference dose (RFD) for oral exposure for barium. Online,* Cincinnati, Ohio, US Environmental Protection Agency, Office of Health and Environmental Assessment, Environmental Criteria and Assessment Office.

VAGT, G.O. (1985) Barite and celesite. In: *Canadian minerals yearbook, 1985: Review and outlook,* Ottawa, Mineral Resources Branch, Department of Energy, Mines and Resources Canada, pp. 10.1-10.4 (Mineral Report No. 34).

VENUGOPAL, B. & LUCKEY, T.D. (1978) *Metal toxicity in mammals: Chemical toxicity of metals and metalloids,* New York, Plenum Press.

VOSS, R.L. & NICOL, H. (1960) Metallic trace elements in tobacco. *Lancet,* II: 435-436.

WALLACH, J. (1978) *Interpretation of diagnostic tests - A handbook synopsis of laboratory medicines,* 3rd ed., Boston, Massachusetts, Little, Brown and Co.

WANG, W. (1986) The effect of river water on phytotoxicity of Ba, Cd and Cr. *Environ. Pollut.,* 11: 193-204.

WANG, P.Y., HAN, J.C., CHANG, P.C., & HAN, Y.M. (1989) Occupational endermatic intoxication of barium - 2 case report. *Chim. J. ind. Hyg. occup. Dis.,* 7: 86-87.

WATERHOUSE, D.F. (1951) Occurrence of barium and strontium in insects. *Aust. J. sci. Res.,* B4: 144-162.

WELLS, R.C. (1937) Analyses of rocks and minerals from the laboratory of the United States Geological Survey, 1914-1936. *US geol. Surv. Bull.,* 878: 134.

WINDHOLZ, M., ed. (1983) *The Merck index,* 10th ed., Rahway, New Jersey, Merck and Co., Inc.

WOLGEMUTH, K. & BROECKER, W.S. (1970) Barium in sea water. *Earth planet. Sci. Lett.,* 8: 372-378.

WONES, R.G., STADLER, B.L., & FROHMAN, L.A. (1990) Lack of effect of drinking water barium on cardiovascular risk factors. *Environ. Health Perspect.,* 85: 1-13.

YARBROUGH, J.D. & O'KELLEY, J.C. (1962) Alkaline earth elements and the avoidance reaction in *Paramecium multimicronucleatum. J. Protozool.,* 9: 132-135.

YOSHIYUKI, T. & YOSHIMASHA, T. (1975) Enhancement of μ-amylase production. Japan. *Kokai*, **160**: 477.

ZDANOWICZ, J.A., FEATHERSTONE, J.D.B., EPSELAND, M.A., & CURZON, M.E.J. (1987) Inhibitory effect of barium on human dental caries prevalence. *Community dent. oral Epidemiol.*, **15**: 6-9.

RESUME ET CONCLUSIONS

1. Résumé

1.1 Identité, état naturel et méthodes d'analyse

Le baryum est un métal alcalino-terreux, de masse atomique relative 137,34 et de numéro atomique 56. Il existe sous la forme de sept isotopes stables présents dans la nature dont le ^{138}Ba est le plus abondant. Le baryum est un métal mou, blanc jaunâtre, fortement électro-positif. Il se combine à l'ammoniac, à l'eau, à l'oxygène, à l'hydrogène, aux halogènes et au soufre en libérant de l'énergie. Il réagit énergiquement avec d'autres métaux pour former des alliages. Dans la nature, on ne le rencontre qu'à l'état combiné, le principal minéral étant la barytine (sulfate de baryum) et la witherite (carbonate de baryum). Le baryum est également présent en petites quantités dans les roches ignées et dans le feldspath et les micas. Il peut également se trouver à l'état naturel dans les combustibles fossiles ainsi que dans l'air, l'eau et le sol.

Certains dérivés du baryum comme l'acétate, le nitrate et le chlorure sont relativement solubles dans l'eau alors que les autres sels tels que le fluorure, le carbonate, l'oxalate, le chromate, le phosphate et le sulfate le sont très peu. A l'exception du sulfate de baryum, la solubilité dans l'eau des sels de baryum augmente à mesure que le pH diminue.

Le prélèvement d'échantillons aqueux ou gazeux pour le dosage du baryum s'effectue de la même manière que pour n'importe quelle autre substance. Les échantillons de sédiments, de boue ou de terre sont séchés au four ou frittés. On procède ensuite à une extraction avec de l'acide chlorhydrique à 1% pour la détermination des éléments en traces et notamment du baryum. Dans le cas des échantillons biologiques, on procède à une congélation ou à une lyophilisation puis on les prépare pour le dosage du baryum par des techniques d'entraînement à sec.

Les méthodes d'analyse les plus fréquemment utilisées sont l'absorption atomique et la spectrométrie d'émission de flamme ou plasma. On a également recours à l'activation neutronique, à la spectrométrie de masse avec dilution isotopique et à la fluorescence X.

1.2 Production, usage et sources d'exposition

La barytine est le minerai dont proviennent presque tous les autres composés du baryum. La production mondiale de barytine était évaluée à 5,7 millions de tonnes en 1985. On utilise le baryum et ses dérivés dans divers produits industriels qui vont des céramiques aux lubrifiants. Ils entrent également dans la fabrication d'alliages et peuvent servir de charges pour le papier, le savon, le caoutchouc, le linoléum. Ils servent aussi à la fabrication de vannes et à l'extinction des feux de radium, d'uranium et de plutonium.

Le baryum résultant d'activités humaines est essentiellement d'origine industrielle. Il peut être émis dans l'environnement à la suite d'activités minières, de raffinage ou de traitement de minerais ou de la fabrication de produits qui en contiennent. Lors de diverses opérations métallurgiques et industrielles, du baryum peut également être rejeté dans les eaux résiduaires. Il peut se déposer sur le sol, par suite de diverses activités humaines, notamment lors du rejet de cendres volantes et de l'enfouissement de boues primaires et secondaires. On estime qu'en 1976, l'extraction et le traitement de la barytine aux Etats-Unis d'Amérique a entraîné le rejet d'environ 3200 tonnes de matières particulaires dans l'atmosphère, les poussières produites par l'utilisation de barytine lors des forages pétroliers et dans l'industrie pétrolière en représentant environ 100 tonnes. En 1972, on estime que l'industrie du baryum a rejeté aux Etats-Unis d'Amérique environ 1200 tonnes de matières particulaires dans l'atmosphère.

Dans l'environnement, le baryum est transporté par l'intermédiaire de l'air, de l'eau et du sol. Dans l'atmosphère, il est présent sous forme de particules dont le transport dépend des conditions atmosphériques et météorologiques. Dans l'eau, ce transport est conditionné par les interactions avec d'autres ions, notamment les ions sulfate, qui régulent et limitent la concentration du baryum. On connaît mal les transformations subies par le baryum ainsi que son transport en milieu aqueux.

Résumé et Conclusions

L'exposition au baryum peut s'effectuer par l'intermédiaire de l'air, de l'eau ou des aliments. On n'est pas très bien renseigné sur les teneurs de l'air en baryum. Aux Etats-Unis d'Amérique, la concentration habituelle est estimée à 0,05 μg/m^3 au plus. On n'a pas constaté de corrélation nette entre la teneur de l'air ambiant en baryum et le degré d'industrialisation, encore que les concentrations soient plus élevées aux alentours des usines métallurgiques.

La présence de baryum dans l'eau de mer, l'eau des rivières et l'eau des puits est attestée et on en trouve également dans les sédiments et les eaux naturelles en contact avec des roches sédimentaires. Le baryum est présent dans presque toutes les eaux superficielles à des concentrations allant jusqu'à 15 000 μg/litre et il contribue à la dureté de l'eau. Dans l'eau des puits, la concentration du baryum dépend de la teneur des roches environnantes en baryum lessivable. L'eau de boisson en contient de 10 à 1000 μg/litre encore que dans certaines régions des Etats-Unis d'Amérique ces concentrations puissent dépasser 10 000 μg/litre. La qualité de l'eau distribuée par les municipalités dépend de celle des eaux de surface et des eaux souterraines et sa teneur en baryum varie dans de larges proportions selon la dureté de l'eau. Des teneurs allant de 1 à 20 μg/litre ont été observées dans l'eau de boisson aux Etats-Unis. Si l'on s'en tient à ces chiffres et pour une consommation de l'ordre de 2 litres par jour, on obtient un apport quotidien de 2 à 40 μg de baryum.

Selon un certain nombre d'études, l'apport quotidien d'origine alimentaire se situe entre 300 et 1770 μg avec d'importantes variations. Il est rare que l'homme consomme des plantes contenant du baryum en quantité importante ou du moins la partie de la plante où le baryum s'accumule. Le noisetier du Brésil constitue une exception, puisque les concentrations observées vont de 1500 à 3000 μg/g. Les tomates et le soja concentrent également le baryum présent dans le sol, le facteur de bio-concentration allant de 2 à 20.

En général le baryum ne s'accumule pas dans les plantes ordinaires en quantité suffisante pour intoxiquer les animaux. Toutefois, on a évoqué la possibilité que les grandes quantités de baryum (jusqu'à 1260 µg/kg) qui s'accumulent dans les légumes, la luzerne et le soja puissent être nocives pour les bovins domestiques.

La teneur en baryum des feuilles de tabac désséchées est de 105 µg/kg en moyenne, la majeure partie restant dans les cendres pendant la combustion. Il n'existe pas de documentation sur la concentration du baryum dans la fumée de tabac.

Les retombées radioactives constituent une autre source d'exposition au baryum. Toutefois, grâce à l'interdiction des essais nucléaires dans l'atmosphère, la quantité de baryum radioactif présent dans l'environnement a diminué.

1.3 Cinétique et surveillance biologique

Un individu moyen (70 kg) renferme environ 22 mg de baryum dans son organisme, qui est en majeure partie (91%) concentré dans les os. On en trouve des traces dans divers tissus ou organes tels que l'aorte, le cerveau, le coeur, le rein, la rate, le pancréas et le poumon. Chez l'homme, la teneur totale en baryum tend à augmenter avec l'âge. Les concentrations dépendent de la zone géographique de résidence des individus. On a trouvé du baryum dans tous les échantillons de tissus provenant d'enfants morts-nés, ce qui donne à penser que cet élément est capable de traverser la barrière placentaire.

Il est difficile d'évaluer l'absorption du baryum après ingestion car elle dépend d'un certain nombre de facteurs. Par exemple, la présence de sulfate dans la nourriture provoque la précipitation du sulfate de baryum. L'expérimentation animale ainsi qu'un certain nombre de données limitées concernant l'homme montrent que le baryum soluble est absorbé au niveau intestinal dans une proportion inférieure à 10% chez l'adulte mais qui peut être supérieure chez les jeunes. Le baryum est rapidement fixé par les glandes salivaires et surrénales, le coeur, les reins, les muqueuses et les vaisseaux sanguins et il finit par aboutir au squelette. En effet, à l'instar du calcium, le baryum s'accumule dans les os. Il se dépose de préférence dans les zones les plus actives de croissance osseuse, principalement à la surface du périoste. L'âge et la privation de nourriture sont également des facteurs importants qui influent sur l'absorption et le dépôt du baryum. Ainsi les rats âgés absorbent moins cet élément et présentent des concentrations osseuses inférieures. Le jeûne augmente en revanche l'absorption du baryum.

Après inhalation, le baryum peut être absorbé au niveau des poumons ou passer directement dans le courant sanguin en traversant la muqueuse nasale. Chez le rat, l'exposition entraîne un dépôt au niveau des os mais lorsqu'elle se poursuit, le dépôt diminue tant au niveau des os qu'au niveau des poumons. Les dérivés insolubles comme le sulfate de baryum s'accumulent dans les poumons et sont lentement éliminés par l'ascenseur muco-ciliaire.

Le baryum est éliminé dans les urines et les matières fécales, dans des proportions qui dépendent de la voie d'administration. Après injection de baryum à des êtres humains, on a constaté qu'en 24 heures, le baryum était éliminé à raison d'environ 20% dans les matières fécales et d'environ 5% dans les urines. Le baryum plasmatique est presque entièrement éliminé du courant sanguin en 24 heures. Chez l'homme et l'animal, l'élimination du baryum après ingestion s'effectue plutôt dans les matières fécales que dans les urines. Après inhalation, le baryum est lentement éliminé des os et par voie de conséquence de l'organisme entier. On estime que la demi-vie biologique du baryum est de 90 à 120 jours chez le rat. Pour assurer une surveillance biologique satisfaisante de l'exposition humaine, il conviendrait de contrôler l'élimination du baryum dans les urines et les matières fécales.

1.4 Effets sur les animaux d'expérience

Chez le rat, on a obtenu des DL_{50} de 118, 250 et 355 respectivement pour le chlorure, le fluorure et le nitrate de baryum. Les effets aigus d'une ingestion de baryum consistent notamment en une salivation, des nausées, de la diarrhée, de la tachycardie, une hypokaliémie, des fibrillations musculaires, une paralysie flasque des muscles squelettiques, une paralysie des muscles respiratoires et une fibrillation ventriculaire. La paralysie des muscles respiratoires et la fibrillation ventriculaire peuvent entraîner la mort. Diverses études ont montré que le baryum perturbait l'action du centre électrogénique de l'automatisme cardiaque. En injectant du baryum par voie intraveineuse à des chiens anesthésiés, on a constaté que ses effets aigus étaient dus à une hypokaliémie importante d'instauration rapide qui pouvait être évitée ou abolie par administration de potassium.

Le baryum provoque une légère irritation cutanée et une forte irritation oculaire chez le lapin.

Des rats qui avaient bu de l'eau du robinet contenant jusqu'à 250 mg de baryum par litre pendant 13 semaines n'ont présenté aucun signe d'intoxication, encore que chez certains groupes on ait noté une réduction du poids relatif des surrénales.

Des rats ayant reçu 10 ou 100 mg de baryum dans leur eau de boisson pendant 16 mois ont présenté une hypertension, mais la tension artérielle n'était pas modifiée à la concentration de 1 mg/litre. L'analyse de la fonction du myocarde au bout de 16 mois à la dose la plus élevée (100 mg de baryum par litre), a révélé que la contractilité et l'excitabilité cardiaque étaient sensiblement modifiées, qu'il y avait des perturbations dans le métabolisme du myocarde et que le système cardio-vasculaire présentait une hypersensibilité au pentobarbital sodique.

Administré à des rats par voie orale ou par inhalation, le carbonate de baryum a excercé des effets nocifs sur leur fonction de reproduction. En outre, on notait un taux de mortalité plus élevé chez les ratons nouveau-nés issus de femelles traitées par du baryum. On possède des preuves limitées d'un pouvoir tératogène du baryum mais aucune donnée concluante quant à sa cancérogénicité.

Du fait de ses propriétés chimiques et physiologiques, le baryum peut entrer en compétition avec le calcium et le remplacer dans les processus où cet élément intervient normalement, notamment la libération de catécholamines par les surrénales et de neurotransmetteurs comme l'acétycholine et la noradrénaline.

On ne possède que peu d'informations sur les effets immunologiques du baryum chez l'animal.

1.5 *Effets sur l'être humain*

On a signalé plusieurs cas d'intoxication consécutifs à l'ingestion de dérivés du baryum. Des doses ne dépassant

Résumé et Conclusions

pas de 0,2 à 0,5 mg de baryum par kg de poids corporel, qui sont généralement consécutives à l'ingestion de chlorure ou de carbonate de baryum, ont provoqué des effets toxiques chez l'adulte. Le tableau clinique d'une intoxication par le baryum se caractérise par une gastro-entérite aiguë, la disparition des réflexes tendineux et l'apparition d'une paralysie musculaire progressive. La paralysie musculaire paraît liée à une hypokaliémie grave. Dans la plupart des cas qui ont été signalés, on a constaté une récupération rapide et sans complications après traitement consistant dans la perfusion de sels de potassium (carbonate ou lactate) et/ou l'administration de sulfate de sodium par voie orale.

Des études épidémiologiques limitées ont été menées pour étudier l'existence d'une relation éventuelle entre la concentration du baryum dans l'eau de boisson et la mortalité par maladies cardiovasculaires; toutefois les résultats obtenus sont irréguliers, et ne permettent pas de conclure.

Chez une population exposée à des fortes concentrations de baryum dans son eau de boisson, on n'a constaté aucune augmentation de l'incidence de l'hypertension, des accidents vasculaires cérébraux ni des maladies cardiaques ou rénales par rapport à un groupe analogue qui était exposé à des concentrations plus faibles. Lors d'une étude de courte durée sur des volontaires, la consommation d'eau de boisson contenant du baryum n'a pas eu d'effets sur la tension artérielle.

On a signalé une augmentation de l'incidence de l'hypertension chez des travailleurs exposés au baryum par rapport à des travailleurs non exposés. Des cas de barytose ont été observés chez des individus exposés de par leur profession à des composés du baryum. Dans un groupe d'étude constitué de travailleurs exposés au baryum et de personnes résidant à proximité d'une décharge où se trouvaient des dérivés du baryum, on a constaté une fréquence accrue de symptômes musculo-squelettiques, d'interventions chirurgicales pour affection gastro-intestinale, de problèmes dermatologiques et de symptômes respiratoires.

On n'a pas constaté d'association concluante entre la teneur de l'eau de boisson en baryum et l'incidence des malformations congénitales. Il n'existe aucune preuve d'une cancérogénicité du baryum.

1.6 Effets sur les êtres vivants dans leur milieu naturel

Le baryum influe directement sur les propriétés physico-chimiques et sur l'infectiosité de plusieurs virus ainsi que sur leur aptitude à se multiplier. Il perturbe également le développement des spores bactériennes en germination et il excerce un certain nombre d'effets sur divers micro-organismes, notamment en inhibant les processus cellulaires.

On connaît mal les effets que le baryum exerce sur les organismes aquatiques. L'exposition de poissons pendant 30 jours à du baryum n'a eu aucun effet sur leur survie. Toutefois, lors d'une étude de 21 jours, on a constaté, chez des daphnies exposées à une dose de 5,8 mg de baryum par litre, des perturbations de leur fonction de reproduction et une moindre croissance. Rien n'indique cependant que la barytine soit toxique pour les animaux marins. Toutefois l'exposition à de grandes quantités de barytine pourrait avoir une influence néfaste sur les colonies de benthos.

Les végétaux et les invertébrés marins pourraient accumuler activement le baryum provenant de l'eau de mer.

2. Conclusions et recommandations

Aux concentrations où il se rencontre habituellement dans l'environnement, le baryum ne présente pas de risque important pour la population dans son ensemble. Toutefois, pour certains sous-groupes et dans des conditions de forte exposition, il faut prendre en compte la possibilité d'effets nocifs sur la santé.

On possède peu de données qui permettraient d'évaluer le risque que le baryum représente sur le plan écologique. Toutefois en s'appuyant sur les données disponibles relatives aux effets toxiques chez les daphnies, il semble que le baryum constitue une menace pour certains organismes aquatiques.

Il est nécessaire de procéder à des études épidémiologiques ainsi qu'à des recherches sur la biodisponibilité du baryum et sur sa toxicité pour le système cardiovasculaire et le système immunitaire; il faudrait également disposer de données complémentaires sur sa toxicité chronique pour la vie aquatique. On aurait besoin de données plus nombreuses sur l'exposition dans les ambiances de travail et sur l'utilisation de marqueurs biologiques afin de pouvoir prendre de meilleures mesures de protection.

EVALUATION DES RISQUES POUR LA SANTE HUMAINE ET EFFETS SUR L'ENVIRONNEMENT

1. Evaluation des risques pour la santé humaine

1.1 Niveaux d'exposition

1.1.1 Population générale

D'après les données en provenance des Etats-Unis d'Amérique, l'apport alimentaire de baryum varie de 300 à 1700 µg/jour. Les valeurs moyennes fournies par deux sources différentes se situent respectivement à 600 et 900 µg/jour.

Des études récentes effectuées aux Etats-Unis d'Amérique indiquent que l'eau de boisson a une teneur en baryum qui varie de 1 à 20 µg/litre. Compte tenu de ces valeurs et en supposant que la consommation quotidienne d'eau de boisson soit de deux litres, l'apport de baryum par cette voie serait de 2 à 40 µg/jour.

Par inhalation, l'apport est estimé à 0,04-3,1 µg/jour.

Au Pays de Galles (Royaume-Uni) on estime que l'apport quotidien de baryum est de 1327 µg (aliments: 1240 µg; eau de boisson: 86 µg; air: 1 µg).

1.1.2 Exposition respiratoire d'origine professionnelle

Chez des ouvriers métallurgistes exposés à des concentrations allant de 0,08 à 1,92 mg/m^3 (moyenne 1,07 mg/m^3) de baryum, on a constaté une forte prévalence de l'hypertension artérielle. Chez un groupe d'ouvriers employés au traitement des minerais de baryum et qui présentaient des symptômes musculo-squelettiques et respiratoires, on a observé une exposition à des concentrations de 0,02 à 1,7 mg/m^3. Chez des soudeurs à l'arc, on a observé des expositions à des concentrations allant de 2,6 à 6,1 mg/m^3. Ce sont les expositions professionnelles les plus fortes qu'on ait signalées mais aucune étude clinique n'a été effectuée.

Evaluation

1.1.3 Exposition aiguë

Des doses ne dépassant pas 0,2 à 0,5 g (3 à 7 mg/kg de poids corporel), telles qu'elles résultent en général de l'ingestion de chlorure ou de carbonate de baryum, entraînent des effets toxiques chez l'adulte. En l'absence de traitement, des doses de 3 à 5 g (40 à 70 mg/kg de poids corporel) ont été mortelles.

1.2 Effets toxiques, relations dose-effet et dose-réponse

L'absorption du baryum dans les voies digestives dépend en grande partie de l'âge et de la solubilité du composé en cause. On pense que le baryum ingéré est absorbé dans une proportion inférieure à 10% chez l'adulte. Toutefois l'absorption peut être sensiblement plus forte chez l'enfant. Après absorption, le baryum pénètre dans le courant sanguin, se fixe dans divers tissus mous et se dépose dans les os. Le métabolisme du baryum est analogue à celui du calcium; toutefois, contrairement à ce dernier, on ne lui connaît aucun rôle biologique. Le baryum peut remplacer le calcium dans de nombreux processus physiologiques et il affecte l'activité nerveuse et musculaire.

Le baryum peut provoquer une légère irritation cutanée et une forte irritation oculaire. On a observé des effets indésirables sur la santé chez des sujets sensibles (malades sous diurétiques) après exposition à du baryum consécutive à l'absorption d'un milieu de contraste baryté en vue d'une radiographie. Plusieurs cas d'intoxication par le baryum ont été signalés. Parmi les symptômes, figurent une gastroentérite aiguë, la disparition des réflexes tendineux et l'apparition d'une paralysie musculaire progressive.

Il n'existe aucune preuve concluante que les dérivés du baryum, à l'exception du chromate, soient cancérogènes pour l'homme. Rien n'indique non plus avec certitude que le baryum ait des effets tératogènes ou embryotoxiques ou des effets nocifs sur la reproduction chez l'homme.

Des études épidémiologiques anciennes, de portée limitée, et concernant les relations entre l'exposition à de faibles teneurs en baryum et la morbidité et la mortalité cardiovasculaires, n'ont pas donné de résultats concluants. Une étude épidémiologique ultérieure n'a pas permis non plus de conclure à un effet du baryum sur la tension artérielle. Lors d'une étude de brève durée au cours de laquelle des volontaires avaient consommé des quantités de plus en plus fortes de baryum allant jusqu'à 10 mg/litre (dans leur eau de boisson), on n'a pas constaté non plus d'effets sur la tension artérielle.

L'inhalation de dérivés du baryum sur les lieux de travail a donné lieu à des cas de barytose. Chez les travailleurs exposés à de fortes concentrations de baryum dans l'atmosphère, on a constaté que l'hypertension artérielle était plus fréquente que chez les ouvriers non exposés. On a fait état, chez le rat exposé à des concentrations de baryum allant jusqu'à 100 mg/litre, d'une augmentation de la pression artérielle systolique.

1.3 Evaluation du risque

Sur la base des publications existantes, on peut conclure qu'aux concentrations où il est généralement présent dans l'eau (spécialement l'eau de boisson), les aliments et l'air ambiant, le baryum ne présente pas de risque important pour la population dans son ensemble. Toutefois dans certains sous-groupes particuliers (les sujets âgés ou qui présentent un déficit de potassium) et dans certaines circonstances particulières (eau fortement chargée en baryum, exposition professionnelle, etc.), il peut y avoir un risque d'effets nocifs sur la santé.

2. Evaluation des effets sur l'environnement

Le baryum est présent dans le sol à une concentration moyenne de 500 μg/g. Dans les océans et les eaux douces, on a mesuré des concentrations allant de 0,04 à 37 μg/litre et de 7,0 à 15 000 μg/litre respectivement. Dans l'air, la concentration du baryum est généralement $\leq$ 0,05 μg/m^3.

Les composés solubles peuvent être transportés dans l'environnement et absorbés par les divers organismes. Le baryum peut s'accumuler dans les différentes parties des végétaux.

D'après certains rapports, le baryum inhiberait la croissance et les processus cellulaires chez les micro-

Evaluation

organismes. On a également constaté qu'il perturbait la germination des spores bactériennes.

On ne dispose pas de renseignements sur les effets nocifs que le baryum exercerait sur les végétaux ou la faune terrestres. Aucun effet toxique n'a été signalé sur les végétaux aquatiques aux concentrations habituellement rencontrées dans l'eau. Pour les poissons d'eau douce, les valeurs de la CL_{50} vont de 46 à 78 mg/litre. On a constaté que des concentrations de baryum égales à 5,8 mg/litre perturbaient la reproduction et la croissance des daphnies.

On manque de données qui permettraient d'évaluer le risque que le baryum constitue pour l'environnement. En se fondant sur les données disponibles concernant les effets toxiques pour les daphnies, il semble que le baryum représente un risque pour certaines populations d'organismes aquatiques.

RECOMMANDATIONS EN VUE D'ETUDES COMPLEMENTAIRES

Il est recommandé de procéder à des recherches complémentaires sur le baryum, à propos de ses effets écologiques et de ses effets sur la santé humaine, dans les secteurs suivants:

- études de biodisponibilité, notamment des mécanismes de solubilisation et de transport;

- études sur l'hypertension et les effets cardiovasculaires au niveau de la population dans son ensemble et des travailleurs exposés de par leur profession; étude des modes d'action;

- études épidémiologiques bien conçues;

- études sur les effets immunologiques du baryum chez l'homme;

- études sur la toxicité sublétale à long terme chez les organismes aquatiques;

- données de surveillance relatives à l'exposition environnementale afin de recenser les secteurs où des mesures de protection sont nécessaires;

- évaluation des indicateurs permettant la détection précoce d'une forte exposition au baryum;

- études sur les marqueurs biologiques (teneur du système pileux et des urines en baryum, taux plasmatique de potassium).

RESUMEN Y CONCLUSIONES

1. Resumen

1.1 Identidad, aparición natural y métodos de análisis

El bario es un metal alcalinotérreo que tiene una masa atómica relativa de 137,34 y un número atómico de 56. Existen siete isótopos estables de aparición natural, de los que el ^{138}Ba es el más abundante. El bario es un metal blando de color blanco amarillento fuertemente electropositivo. Se combina con el amoniaco, el agua, el oxígeno, el hidrógeno, los halógenos y el azufre, liberando energía en esas reacciones. También reacciona fuertemente con los metales para constituir aleaciones metálicas. En la naturaleza, el bario aparece sólo en forma combinada, siendo las principales formas minerales la barita (sulfato de bario) y la witherita (carbonato de bario). El bario se halla también en pequeñas cantidades en las rocas ígneas y en el feldespato y las micas. Puede encontrarse como componente natural de los combustibles fósiles y se halla en el aire, el agua y el suelo.

Ciertos compuestos de bario, como el acetato, el nitrato y el cloruro, son relativamente hidrosolubles, mientras que las sales de fluoruro, carbonato, oxalato, cromato, fosfato y sulfato presentan una solubilidad muy baja. Con la excepción del sulfato de bario, la solubilidad en agua de las sales de bario aumenta al disminuir el pH.

El muestreo del bario en los medios acuosos y gaseosos se realiza del mismo modo que en el caso de cualquier otro material. Las muestras de sedimentos, barro y tierra se desecan en horno o se sinterizan. Después se extraen las muestras con HCl al 1% para el análisis de los oligoelementos, incluido el bario. Las muestras biológicas se congelan o liofilizan y se preparan para el análisis del bario utilizando procedimientos de lavado en seco.

Los métodos de análisis empleados más corrientemente son la absorción atómica y la espectrometría de llama y emisión del plasma. También se utilizan la activación neutrónica, la espectrometría de masa por dilución de isótopos y la fluorescencia con rayos X.

1.2 Producción, utilizaciones y fuentes de exposición

El mineral barita es el material bruto del que se extraen casi todos los demás compuestos de bario. La producción mundial de barita se estimó en 1985 en 5,7 millones de toneladas. El bario y sus compuestos se emplean en distintos productos industriales que comprenden desde la cerámica hasta los lubricantes. Se utiliza en la fabricación de aleaciones, como cargador para papel, jabón, caucho y linóleo, en la fabricación de válvulas y como extintor en los incendios provocados por radio, uranio y plutonio.

Las fuentes antropogénicas de bario son fundamentalmente industriales. Las emisiones pueden deberse a la minería, el refino o el tratamiento de minerales de bario y a la fabricación de productos de bario. El bario aparece también en las aguas residuales procedentes de la metalurgia y de otras industrias. La deposición en el suelo puede deberse a las actividades humanas, que comprenden la eliminación de cenizas y el empleo de fangos primarios y secundarios en el relleno de tierras. Se ha calculado que en 1976, la minería y el tratamiento del mineral barita en los Estados Unidos de América liberaron unas 3200 toneladas de partículas en el aire y que los polvos fugitivos procedentes del uso de barita en la perforación petrolífera y en industrias conexas representaron alrededor de 100 toneladas de partículas. En 1972, en los Estados Unidos de América, la industria química del bario desprendió alrededor de 1200 toneladas de partículas en la atmósfera.

El transporte ambiental del bario se produce por el aire, el agua y el suelo. El bario atmosférico consiste en partículas cuyo transporte está regulado por las condiciones atmosféricas y meteorológicas normales. El transporte del bario por el agua está sometido a la interacción con otros iones, en particular el sulfato, que regula y limita la concentración de bario. Se dispone de escasa información acerca de las transformaciones y el transporte de bario por el agua.

La exposición al bario puede producirse por el aire, el agua o los alimentos. No se poseen datos suficientes sobre las concentraciones de bario en el aire. En los Estados Unidos de América se ha calculado que la concentración habitual es de 0,05 $\mu g/m^3$ o menos. No se ha observado una correlación neta entre las concentraciones ambientales de bario en el aire y la amplitud de la industrialización, aunque pueden producirse mayores concentraciones alrededor de las fundiciones.

Se ha probado la presencia de bario en el agua de mares, ríos y manantiales, y se ha hallado también en sedimentos y aguas naturales en contacto con rocas sedimentarias. El bario se encuentra en casi todas la aguas superficiales en concentraciones de hasta 15 000 μg/litro y contribuye a la dureza del agua. La concentración del bario en el agua de manantial depende del contenido de bario lixiviable de las rocas. El agua potable contiene 10-1000 μg/litro, aunque se ha observado que el agua de ciertas regiones de los Estados Unidos de América presenta concentraciones superiores a 10 000 μg/litro. Los suministros municipales de agua dependen de la calidad de las aguas de superficie y freáticas y, en función de la dureza, contienen una amplia gama de concentraciones de bario. Los estudios efectuados en los Estados Unidos de América muestran que las concentraciones en el agua potable varían entre 1 y 20 μg/litro. Basándose en esos datos y suponiendo un consumo de 2 litros por día, la ingesta diaria sería de 2-40 μg de bario.

En varios estudios se ha calculado una ingesta alimentaria diaria de 300 a 1770 μg, con amplias variaciones. Las personas rara vez comen plantas en las que se halle el bario en concentraciones notables o partes de la planta en las que se acumule el bario. El nogal del Brasil es una excepción, pues se han hallado concentraciones de 1500-3000 $\mu g/g$. También se sabe que los tomates y las habas de soja concentran el bario del suelo, con un factor de bioconcentración comprendido entre 2 y 20.

Por lo general, el bario no se acumula en las plantas corrientes en cantidades suficientes para que sea tóxico para los animales. Sin embargo, se ha señalado que las altas cantidades de bario (hasta 1260 mg/kg) acumuladas en las verduras, el alfalfa y las habas de soja pueden producir problemas en el ganado bovino.

El contenido de bario de las hojas de tabaco secas alcanza un promedio de 105 mg/kg y es probable que la mayor parte permanezca en la ceniza en el curso de la combustión. No se han señalado las concentraciones de bario en el humo del tabaco.

Otra fuente de exposición al bario es la lluvia radiactiva. Sin embargo, la adopción de tratados que prohíben las pruebas en la atmósfera ha reducido la cantidad de bario radiactivo presente en el medio.

1.3 Cinética y vigilancia biológica

La persona media (70 kg) contiene unos 22 mg de bario, hallándose la mayor parte (91%) en el esqueleto. Se encuentran cantidades infinitesimales en varios órganos como la aorta, el cerebro, el corazón, los riñones, el bazo, el páncreas y los pulmones. El bario total del organismo humano tiende a aumentar con la edad. Las concentraciones observadas en el organismo dependen de la situación geográfica del individuo. También se ha encontrado bario en todas las muestras de recién nacidos, lo que permite pensar que atraviesa la placenta.

Es difícil evaluar la captación del bario ingerido porque distintos factores influyen en la absorción. Por ejemplo, la presencia de sulfato en los alimentos se debe a la precipitación del sulfato de bario. Los estudios efectuados en animales de experimentación y los limitados datos obtenidos en personas muestran que el bario soluble se absorbe por el intestino hasta el < 10% en los adultos, pero más en los jóvenes. La captación se produce rápidamente en las glándulas salivales y suprarrenales, el corazón, los riñones, las mucosas y los vasos sanguíneos y, por último, el esqueleto. Igual que el calcio, el bario se acumula en los huesos. Se deposita de preferencia en las zonas más activas del crecimiento óseo, y sobre todo en las superficies periósticas. Entre otros factores importantes en la absorción y la deposición figuran la edad y las restricciones alimentarias. Las ratas de edad avanzada presentan una disminución de la absorción y de las concentraciones óseas de bario. El ayuno desencadena un aumento de la absorción de bario.

El bario inhalado puede absorberse por el el pulmón o directamente por la mucosa nasal pasando a la corriente sanguínea. En las ratas, la exposición da lugar a la deposición en los huesos, pero la exposición continua origina una disminución de la deposición en los huesos y los pulmones. Los compuestos insolubles, como el sulfato bárico, se acumulan en los pulmones y se eliminan lentamente por la acción de los cilios.

El bario se elimina por la orina y la heces, en tasas que varían conforme a la vía de administración. Una dosis de bario inyectada al hombre se elimina en 24 horas en un 20% aproximadamente por las heces yen alrededor del 5% por la orina. El bario plasmático queda eliminado casi por completo de la corriente sanguínea en 24 horas. La eliminación del bario ingerido en el hombre y los animales se produce por las heces más que por la orina. Tras la exposición por inhalación, se produce una lenta eliminación del bario de los huesos y por consiguiente de todo el organismo. En las ratas se ha calculado que la semivida biológica del bario es de 90-120 días. Para efectuar una vigilancia biológica apropiada de la exposición humana debe observarse la eliminación del bario por la orina y las heces.

1.4 Efectos en los animales de experimentación

En la rata, los valores de la DL_{50} oral son de 118, 250 y 355 en los casos del cloruro, el fluoruro y el nitrato de bario, respectivamente. Entre los efectos agudos de la ingestión de bario figuran los siguientes: salivación, náuseas, diarrea, taquicardia, hipopotasemia, calambres, parálisis fláccida de la musculatura esquelética, parálisis de los músculos respiratorios y fibrilación ventricular. La parálisis de los músculos respiratorios y la fibrilación ventricular pueden conducir a la muerte. En varios estudios se ha demostrado el efecto nocivo del bario sobre el automatismo ventricular y las corrientes marcapasos del corazón. La inyección intravenosa de bario a perros anestesiados muestra que esos efectos agudos se deben a la aparición rápida de una hipopotasemia notable y pueden evitarse o contrarrestarse por la administración de potasio.

El bario produce irritación moderada de la piel e intensa de los ojos en el conejo.

En ratas que ingirieron agua del grifo que contenía hasta 250 mg de bario/litro durante 13 semanas, no se observaron signos de toxicidad, aunque algunos grupos presentaron un descenso del peso relativo de las suprarrenales.

Las ratas que recibieron 10 o 100 mg de bario/litro en su agua de beber durante 16 meses presentaron hipertensión, pero una concentración de 1 mg/litro no ocasionó cambio alguno de la tensión arterial. Los análisis de la función miocárdica a los 16 meses (dosis de 100 mg de bario/litro) mostraron alteraciones significativas de la contractilidad y la excitabilidad del corazón, alteraciones metabólicas del miocardio e hipersensibilidad del sistema cardiovascular al pentobarbital sódico.

En las ratas, la administración oral o la inhalación de carbonato bárico influyeron desfavorablemente en la reproducción. Además la tasa de mortalidad fue mayor en las crías recién nacidas de madres tratadas con bario. Algunos datos muestran la teratogenicidad del bario, pero no se dispone de indicios concluyentes de cancerogenicidad.

El bario posee propiedades químicas y fisiológicas que le permiten competir con el calcio y sustituirlo en los procesos en los que este elemento actúa normalmente de mediador, en particular en los relacionados con la liberación de catecolaminas adrenales y de neurotransmisores, como la acetilcolina y la noradreladina.

Se dispone de información limitada acerca de los efectos inmunológicos del bario en los animales.

1.5 *Efectos en la especie humana*

Se han señalado varios casos de intoxicación por ingestión de compuestos de bario. Se ha observado que dosis de bario tan bajas como 0,2-0,5 mg/kg de peso corporal, resultantes en general de la ingestión de cloruro o carbonato de bario, producen efectos tóxicos en el hombre. El cuadro clínico producido por la intoxicación por bario comprende gastroenteritis aguda, pérdida de los reflejos profundos con comienzo de parálisis muscular, y parálisis muscular progresiva. La parálisis muscular parece guardar relación con la hipopotasemia intensa. En la mayoría de los casos notificados se produjo una recuperación rápida y sin problemas después del tratamiento consistente en la perfusión de sales de potasio (carbonato o lactato) y/o en la administración oral de sulfato sódico.

Se han realizado estudios epidemiológicos limitados para estudiar la posible relación existente entre las concentraciones de bario en el agua potable y la mortalidad cardiovascular, pero los resultados han sido incoherentes y nada concluyentes.

No se han observado aumentos de la incidencia de la hipertensión arterial, los accidentes cerebrovasculares o las enfermedades cardiacas y renales en una población expuesta a altas concentraciones de bario en el agua de beber, en comparación con un grupo análogo expuesto a menores niveles. En un estudio a corto plazo en voluntarios humanos, el consumo de bario en el agua de beber no influyó en la tensión arterial.

Se ha comunicado un aumento de la incidencia de la hipertensión en trabajadores expuestos al bario, en comparación con los no expuestos. Se ha observado la aparición de baritosis en personas expuestas profesionalmente a compuestos de bario. En un grupo estudiado formado por trabajadores expuestos al bario y personas que vivían cerca de un lugar rellenado con productos que contenían bario se observó una mayor prevalencia de síntomas musculoesqueléticos, intervenciones quirúrgicas gastrointestinales, problemas cutáneos y síntomas respiratorios.

No se ha observado ninguna asociación concluyente entre la concentración de bario del agua de beber y la incidencia de malformaciones congénitas. No hay indicios de que el bario sea carcinógeno.

1.6 Efectos en los seres vivos del medio ambiente

El bario influye directamente en las propiedades fisicoquímicas y en la infecciosidad de varios virus, así como en su capacidad de multiplicación. Afecta también al desarrollo de esporas bacterianas en germinación y ejerce distintos efectos específicos sobre diferentes microorganismos, incluida la inhibición de los procesos celulares.

Se dispone de escasa información sobre los efectos del bario en los seres vivos acuáticos. No se han observado efectos en la supervivencia de peces sometidos a una exposición de 30 días de duración. Sin embargo, en un estudio de 21 días se observaron alteraciones de la reproducción y reducción del crecimiento en dafnidos empleando dosis de 5,8 mg de bario/litro. No se han recogido indicios que muestren que la barita es tóxica para los animales marinos. Sin embargo, la exposición a la barita en grandes concentraciones puede influir desfavorablemente en la colonización producida por la fauna béntica.

Los vegetales y los invertebrados marinos pueden acumular activamente bario procedente del agua del mar.

2. Conclusiones y recomendaciones

En las concentraciones halladas normalmente en nuestro medio ambiente, el bario no plantea ningún riesgo importante para la población en general. Sin embargo, en el caso de determinadas subpoblaciones y en condiciones de alta exposición al bario, deben tomarse en consideración las posibilidades de efectos adversos en la salud.

Se dispone de escasos datos para evaluar el riesgo del bario para el medio ambiente. Sin embargo, basándose en la información disponible sobre los efectos tóxicos del bario en los dáfnidos, parece que puede representar un riesgo para las poblaciones de ciertos seres vivos acuáticos.

Se necesitan estudios epidemiológicos, investigaciones sobre la biodisponibilidad y la toxicidad cardiovascular e inmunitaria, e información adicional sobre la toxicidad acuática crónica. Para establecer mejores medidas de protección se requieren más datos sobre la exposición en el lugar de trabajo y el uso de biomarcadores.

Evaluación

EVALUACION DE LOS RIESGOS PARA LA SALUD HUMANA Y DE LOS EFECTOS SOBRE EL MEDIO AMBIENTE

1. Evaluación de los riesgos para la salud humana

1.1 Niveles de exposición

1.1.1 Población general

La ingesta alimentaria de bario, basada en datos procedentes de los Estados Unidos de América, es de 300 a 1700 µg/día. Los valores medios notificados por dos fuentes distintas son de 600 y 900 µg/día.

Recientes estudios estadounidenses muestran que las concentraciones de bario en el agua potable van de 1 a 20 µg/litro. Basándose en esa gama y suponiendo un consumo diario de dos litros de agua potable, la ingesta de bario en el agua de beber sería de 2-40 µg/día.

La entrada de bario por la inhalación se calcula en 0,04 a 3,1 µg/día.

Según las estimaciones efectuadas en Gales (Reino Unido), la toma diaria total de bario es de 1327 µg (alimentos: 1240 µg; agua de beber: 86 µg; aire: 1 µg).

1.1.2 Exposición al aire del medio laboral

La exposición de los trabajadores en la industria de aleaciones metálicas a concentraciones comprendidas entre 0,08 y 1,92 mg/m^3 (media: 1,07 mg/m^3) da lugar a una elevada prevalencia de la hipertensión. En un grupo de trabajadores de transformación de mineral de bario que presentaban síntomas musculoesqueléticos y respiratorios se observaron exposiciones de 0,02 a 1,7 mg/m^3. En soldadores con arco de acero se han medido exposiciones a concentraciones comprendidas entre 2,2 a 6,1 mg/m^3. Son las mayores concentraciones ocupacionales que se han notificado, pero no se realizaron estudios médicos.

1.1.3 Exposiciones agudas

Se ha observado que dosis de bario tan bajas como 0,2-0,5 g (3-7 mg/kg de peso corporal), resultantes en general de la ingestión de cloruro o carbonato de bario, provocan efectos tóxicos en personas adultas. En casos sin tratar, dosis de 3-5 g (40-70 mg/kg de peso corporal) resultaron mortales.

1.2 Efectos tóxicos; relaciones dosis-efecto y dosis-respuesta

La absorción de bario por el tracto gastrointestinal depende en gran parte de la edad y de la solubilidad del producto. Se cree que en los adultos se absorbe menos del 10% del bario ingerido. Ahora bien, la absorción puede ser notablemente mayor en los niños. El bario absorbido penetra en la corriente sanguínea y en varios tejidos blandos y se deposita en el esqueleto; el metabolismo del bario es análogo al del calcio, pero la diferencia estriba en que el bario no tiene ninguna función biológica conocida. El bario puede sustituir al calcio en numerosos procesos fisiológicos y afecta a la actividad nerviosa y muscular.

El contacto con bario puede producir irritación moderada de la piel e intensa de los ojos. Se han observado efectos nocivos en personas sensibles (por ejemplo, enfermos sometidos a diuresis) tras la exposición al bario como medio de examen radiológico. Se han registrado algunos casos de intoxicación por bario. Entre los síntomas figuran la gastroenteritis aguda, la pérdida de reflejos profundos con comienzo de parálisis muscular, y la parálisis muscular progresiva.

No hay datos concluyentes en el sentido de que los productos de bario, con excepción del cromato, sean carcinógenos en el hombre. Tampoco puede afirmarse que el bario produzca efectos en la reproducción, embriotóxicos o teratógenos en la especie humana.

Los limitados estudios epidemiológicos iniciales que establecían una relación entre la exposición a concentraciones bajas de bario y la morbilidad y mortalidad cardiovascular eran incoherentes y nada concluyentes. En un estudio epidemiológico ulterior no se encontró ningún

Evaluación

dato decisivo que pusiera de manifiesto efectos del bario en la tensión arterial. Tampoco se observaron esos efectos en un estudio a corto plazo en el que un grupo de voluntarios consumió concentraciones crecientes de bario hasta de 10 mg/litro de agua de beber.

El bario inhalado en el lugar de trabajo ha dado lugar a baritosis. La prevalencia de la hipertensión en trabajadores expuestos a concentraciones altas de bario transportado por el aire fue claramente superior a la observada en trabajadores que no sufrieron esa exposición. Se señaló un aumento de la tensión arterial sistólica relacionado con la dosis en ratas expuestas a concentraciones de bario de hasta 100 mg/litro.

1.3 Evaluación del riesgo

Basándose en las publicaciones disponibles, puede llegarse a la conclusión de que la salud de la población general no corre ningún riesgo significativo por la acción del bario en las concentraciones halladas habitualmente en el agua (especialmente el agua de beber), los alimentos y el aire ambiental. Sin embargo, en el caso de determinadas subpoblaciones (ancianos o personas con deficiencia de potasio) y en circunstancias particulares (concentración elevada en el agua, exposición profesional, etc.) puede haber posibilidades de efectos adversos para la salud.

2. Evaluación de los efectos sobre el medio ambiente

El bario se halla en el suelo a una concentración media de 500 $\mu g/g$. Se han medido concentraciones de 0,04 a 37,0 $\mu g/litro$ y de 7,0 a 15 000 $\mu g/litro$ en las aguas oceánicas y dulces, respectivamente. Las concentraciones de bario en el aire son en general de $\leq$ 0,05 $\mu g/m^3$.

Los compuestos de bario solubles pueden transportarse por el medio ambiente y ser absorbidos por los seres vivos. El bario puede acumularse en distintas partes de las plantas.

Se ha señalado que el bario inhibe el crecimiento y los procesos celulares de los microorganismos. Se ha observado también que influye en el desarrollo de las esporas bacterianas en germinación.

No se han hallado datos sobre los efectos adversos del bario en las plantas terrestres o los animales silvestres. En las plantas acuáticas no se han registrado efectos tóxicos debidos al bario en las concentraciones habituales en el agua. Los valores de CL_{50} para los peces de agua dulce son de 46 a 78 mg/litro. Se ha observado que las concentraciones de bario de 5,8 mg/litro alteran la reproducción y el crecimiento de los dáfnidos.

Faltan datos para evaluar el riesgo que supone el bario para el medio ambiente. Basándose en la información disponible sobre los efectos tóxicos en los dáfnidos, parece que el bario puede representar un riesgo para las poblaciones de ciertos seres vivos acuáticos.

RECOMENDACIONES PARA ULTERIORES ESTUDIOS

Se recomiendan investigaciones ulteriores sobre el bario en los siguientes sectores de los efectos en el medio ambiente y la salud humana:

- estudios de biodisponibilidad, que comprendan los mecanismos de solubilización y transporte;

- estudios sobre hipertensión/enfermedades cardiovasculares, que abarquen la población general y los trabajadores expuestos por razones profesionales, y mecanismos de acción conexos;

- estudios epidemiológicos bien planeados;

- estudios sobre los efectos inmunológicos del bario en el hombre;

- estudios sobre la toxicidad acuática subletal a largo plazo;

- datos de vigilancia sobre la exposición ambiental para determinar los sectores en los que se necesitan medidas protectoras;

- evaluación de indicadores iniciales de alta tasa de exposición al bario; estudios de marcadores biológicos (por ejemplo, contenido de bario en el pelo y la orina, concentraciones de potasio sérico).